E. Schorsch G. Galedary A. Haag
M. Hauch H. Lohse

Sex Offenders

Dynamics and Psychotherapeutic Strategies

Translated from the German
by Tom Todd and Jane Wiebel

Foreword by Anke Erhardt

Springer-Verlag Berlin Heidelberg New York
London Paris Tokyo Hong Kong

Authors:

Prof. Dr. med. Eberhard Schorsch
Dipl. Psych. Gerlinde Galedary
Dipl. Psych. Margret Hauch
Dipl. Psych. Hartwig Lohse
Abteilung für Sexualforschung

Dr. med. Antje Haag
Abteilung für Psychosomatik und Psychotherapie

Universitätskrankenhaus Eppendorf
Martinistraße 52, 2000 Hamburg 20, FRG

Translators:

Tom Todd
Chr.-Förster-Straße 20, 2000 Hamburg 20, FRG

Dr. Jane Wiebel
Isestraße 129, 2000 Hamburg 13, FRG

Title of the Original German Edition:
Perversion als Straftat. Dynamik und Psychotherapie

ISBN-13:978-3-540-51042-0

ISBN-13:978-3-540-51042-0 e-ISBN-13:978-3-642-74690-1
DOI: 10.1007/978-3-642-74690-1

2119/3140-543210 - Printed on acid-free paper

Foreword

This book focuses on the treatment of men who have committed either sexually offensive acts (such as indecent exposure to women or children, phone harassment, or voyeurism) or sexual crimes (such as rape or sexual acts against children). Not enough research has been done on the therapeutic rehabilitation of sex offenders, and the issue is therefore poorly understood. For the most part, sex offenders are only seen in the context of the criminal justice system, i.e., punishment and imprisonment. Relatively little research has been reported on clinical treatment strategies, which have ranged from surgical castration, to hormonal suppression of sexual drive with antiandrogens, and more frequently to behavioral therapy approaches based on models of learning theories. Generally, clinicians and researchers shy away from working with these people because of their skepticism of whether anything at all will be effective, and their fear of the more basic conflict over whether this person as a clinical patient rather than a criminal best dealt with within the legal system.

This book is unique in that it reports on a program that has applied a multifaceted psychotherapeutic approach to dealing with sex offenders, and specifically includes dynamic principles of the patient-therapist relationship. The authors give a detailed account of their work with 86 men with sexually deviant behavior. They describe a creative treatment model which is eclectic, comprehensive and tailored to this patient population's needs. It includes: help in coping with everyday life, interventions with current crises, behavior therapy for definable problem areas, and interpretation and confrontation within the patient-therapist relationship. This approach is not only unique because it includes components of several different treatment modalities, but also because it is pragmatic and flexible. For instance, while most patients were treated with once-a-week individual outpatient sessions, at times the authors included inpatient admissions, couple therapy, and groups.

Another strength and important feature of this book is that it does not only report on a well-defined treatment model but deals with it within the framework of research. The patient group was compared to a waiting-list group. The success of treatment was rated according to clearly defined guidelines and was judged by independent raters. The assessment of effectiveness is based on concrete criteria, such as symptom recurrence, social integration, and a more global personality integration index. In addition, it includes a short- and long-term follow-up component.

The authors are members of a well-known department of sex research at the University of Hamburg Medical School in West Germany. The work of that department, which has a record of pioneering research studies, is internationally known and highly respected. This book will be of great interest to clinicians who work with patients who have sexual problems or who have commited sexual crimes. Furthermore, it provides a conceptual framework for the large number of psychologists, psychiatrists, and social workers who are not specialists in this area, but who occasionally deal with individuals who have sexual problems. The authors offer guidelines for clinicians and suggest that it more effective for this group of patients not to be seen exclusively by experts, but also by therapists with more general practices or services.

Apart from providing innovative information, the book is interesting to read and includes pivotal case reports and examples. It fills a gap in an under-researched area and offers a systematic treatment approach that is effective as well as humane.

Anke A. Ehrhardt, Ph. D.
Professor of Clinical Psychology
Department of Psychiatry
Columbia University, College of Physicians and Surgeons
New York, NY

Preface

The subject of this book is psychotherapy for men who have come into conflict with the law because of their perverse symptoms. The focus lies on perversions which constitute an illegal form of behaviour so that performing them is a *criminal act*. This particular aspect has for the most part been neglected in psychodynamic literature on perversions. Whenever sexual perversions are viewed mainly from the psychotherapeutic angle, they tend to be regarded as secret phantasies or private performances. Seen from the point of view of the individual involved, the phenomenon of perversion has emerged as a creative achievement on the part of the ego; it has frequently been admired as a minor work of art defending the ego, and the result has often been that the therapist decided to leave this subtle construction untouched. The perspective changes radically once the sexual delinquent becomes the focus of attention; as a rule, research then no longer adopts a psychodynamic approach to understanding perversion. A perverse act is judged rather than understood and no doubt is left as to the necessity of symptom removal. In this book we shall primarily consider perversion as a criminal act and not as a work of art. It was the continual confrontation with such problems in the outpatient clinic at the Department of Sex Research, along with our involvement in writing forensic reports, which led us to carry out this research project. In the long run it is difficult to reconcile one's role as a consultant in criminal proceedings with a therapeutic approach and attitude; the broader one's understanding of the psychodynamics of a sexual offence, the more urgent becomes the pressure to draw therapeutic conclusions.

The special value of our research work lies in the fact that, as well as single case studies, we systematically examined a large group of patients (86), looking into diagnostic criteria and therapeutic processes. This is new in psychodynamic literature. In the scattered cases where therapy with a larger group of sex offenders has been reported, the approach has always been a behaviourist one, in which a therapy concept was presented and applied to these patients. The results of such studies only offered insight into the efficacy of a particular therapeutic technique or programme for these patients. In this book, however, we do not intend to assess how well a particular therapy programme works, but enquire rather to what extent each of these patients seen as an individual is accessible to psychotherapy.

With this book we hope to convey something of what we learned and gained while working on this project and want above all to encourage other therapists to take up work with these patients.

Hamburg, Spring 1990 The Authors

Contents

1 Introduction

1.1 Sexual Delinquency and Therapy: The Current State of Affairs

Although we know in theory that a criminal act is often an acting out of inner conflicts and that sexual deviancy in particular is one of a series of symptoms of psychic disorder, this is generally ignored in psychotherapeutic *practice*. Hardly anybody feels they are competent or responsible for carrying out therapy with these patients.

Patients suffering from sexual deviancy problems usually only come into contact with psychiatrists once they have broken the law: either through an expertise for the court or when they have been assigned to a psychiatric state hospital by court order. Giving *medical evidence* is conceived primarily as a diagnostic process; therapeutic perspectives are discussed at best theoretically but usually do not fall within the jurisdiction of the court itself.

Patients committed to psychiatric state hospitals have, as a rule, little chance of obtaining therapy. On the one hand the institutional situation and staffing allows no free space for any therapeutic efforts; on the other the psychiatrists in these institutions frequently lack the appropriate pyschotherapeutic training.

The situation in *prison* is by no means better. The senselessness of gaol sentences, especially for sexual delinquents whose inner problems are frequently increased rather than diminished during imprisonment so that relapses become inevitable, is also recognized and regretted by the legal authorities.

The burden of the situation falls on the offenders. All they can expect from the psychiatrists is either a diagnostic examination, usually including moral labels, or, as in most cases, being kept in custody. They can hardly expect any help from psychotherapists as they are as a rule quite unfamiliar with the problems involved. In fact what happens is that sex offenders, once the court has ordered treatment for them, are sent from one therapist to the next and only in the rarest cases do they find an opportunity to undergo psychotherapy.

The only therapeutic concepts developed by psychiatrists and still applied on a large scale are *somatic methods of treatment*.

1. The most common is suppression of sexual drive using *anti-androgens*. These work by competing with and inhibiting the androgen receptors and cause reduction or loss of libido and potency for the duration of medication, depending on the dosage. This is accompanied by a halt in the production of

sperm (infertility); both ejaculation and the intensity of orgasm become weaker. As far as we know, these effects are reversible, and the undesirable effects in adults do not exceed acceptable limits (see review in Neumann and Steinbeck 1974).

Because of the almost complete lack of therapeutic facilities for sexual delinquents, anti-androgens were enthusiastically welcomed. In the Federal Republic of Germany (FRG) they have been propagated as a panacea in this field. Criminal proceedings against a recidivist delinquent nowadays hardly ever end without anti-androgen treatment being considered. Misuse and blind application are common. This does not mean that we wish to question the general value of anti-androgens. It must be emphasized, however, that this treatment concentrates merely on the symptom in the sense that at least the symptom can be got rid of. Unless coupled with psychotherapeutic treatment of the underlying problems this medication, as Petri (1980) emphasized, only offers a pseudosolution and moreover brings with it the risk of making problems and symptoms chronic.

2. The mutilating effects of *surgical castration* have more in common with getting even with these people than with therapy. We shall show that pronounced masculinity problems lie behind many sex offences and that, psychoanalytically speaking, castration anxieties play a large role. Surgical castration means that this wound is literally opened up further with the scalpel or, if the patient requested surgery, that the surgeon acts out the patient's longing to be punished. This is also true, with some exceptions, of anti-androgen treatment. Castration used to be carried out quite frequently. It was legitimated by old investigations which quoted a relapse rate of between 2% and 5% (e.g. Langelüddeke 1963). More recent, critical investigations (Heim 1977) on both relapse rates and the earlier positive assessments of the effects and side effects come to much more sceptical conclusions. A critical analysis of the castration issue is available in Sigusch (1978). Surgical castration should have become a relic of the past once anti-androgens, which have a similar although reversible effect, had been introduced.

3. Particularly in the 1970s a lot was heard about *stereotactic brain surgery* as a method of treatment for sexual deviations. This involved selective surgical disconnection of an area in the diencephalon in which a so-called "sex centre" was allegedly located. The operation was supposed to induce a change in sexual behaviour and/or a reduction of "sexual drive". A critical review of the results and their documentation showed that, quite apart from the ethical dubiousness of surgery aimed at altering the psyche, nothing could be said about the reliability of this method: the theoretical foundation is unclear, effects and side effects have not been adequately investigated (Rieber et al. 1976). Sigusch (1977) and Schorsch and Schmidt (1979) have published detailed criticisms of this form of intervention. A Federal Health Authority commission set up by the Federal government to examine this issue came to generally critical and sceptical conclusions (Fülgraff and Barbey 1978). Following a few setbacks after the initial excitement this method caused, little has been heard of it since; as far as

we know it is nowadays no longer applied to sexual delinquents in West Germany.

All these somatic methods are based on purely *symptom-oriented pragmatism* which lacks theoretical backing and fails to do justice to the meaning of sexuality and the formation of sexually deviant symptoms. Nor can this shortcoming be remedied by the relatively high success quota which is always reported. In the case of therapy for psychological problems in general, i.e. anxieties, crises, conflicts, helplessness, it is very tempting but extremely problematic to adopt a method whose only criterion is that it removes the symptom. This approach, which can be easily linked to a calculation of the relative costs and effects in financial terms, harbours the danger of losing sight of the individual human being and the human dimensions - even though the patient may be a social "failure" and may have a damaging effect on others. The real intention, especially behind the medical methods mentioned, is to cut off one important area of experience - sexuality - which inevitably means an impoverishment in the quality of the patient's life.

In Sect. 1.3 we shall present the results of our *review of the literature on psychotherapy for these patient groups*. In summary, one can say that apart from one or two isolated studies only very few systematic investigations exist; these derive mainly from behaviour therapy and show a preference for aversion techniques which have a punitive nature, just like the medical interventions. Putting things bluntly, this essentially means that the only alternative left for sexual delinquents is punishment - whether legal, medical or psychotherapeutic; and the counteraggression revealed in such procedures is unmistakeable.

The lack of careful scientific thought given to psychotherapy for sex offenders is paralleled by the way therapists and therapy institutions ignore or neglect these patients. The psychotherapists (and many of the patients, too) are frightened of getting involved and justify this with weak arguments.

1. The repeated categorical assertion that patients with a perversion do not "really" *suffer* any distress, because of the pleasurable feelings they have as a result of the symptom, and are therefore not really motivated for therapy has left its mark in the scientific literature. This view is used to legitimate a general fear of getting involved with these patients and therefore leaves psychotherapists little opportunity for discovering the true state of affairs. "I have hardly seen a single perverse person who - besides satisfying his instinctual desires - did not suffer from his perversion, from the allied loss of his ability to love and the real threat and isolation linked to it" (Riemann 1968). As with many kinds of symptoms, it seems to us more appropriate to view and discuss momentary desire and satisfaction, as far as they are experienced at all intensely in a sex offence, in the wider context of secondary gain. We have by no means forgotten that the key notion "motivation for therapy" presents special problems for these patients, which distinguishes them from other psychotherapy patients. We shall discuss these problems in detail in Sect. 4.2 and come to the conclusion

that the motivation concept and the ideas it implies have to be revised. An apparent lack of motivation does not provide grounds for refusing to offer therapy.

2. Another widespread argument used to reject psychotherapy for delinquents is that it is only feasible if strictly voluntary and that, for example, a pending trial or a *court order for treatment* constitutes a counterindication. Goudsmit and Reicher (1980), who have probably had the most practical experience in psychotherapy with sex offenders, consider it "inhumane" to refuse a patient for this reason. Petri (1980) believes that such external pressure actually benefits therapy (as do Bronisch et al. 1983; Giese and Kober 1983). Our results also showed that outside pressure presents at least no hindrance to therapy (see Sect. 4.5.2.6.1, Table 26). Nor have we by any means ignored the difficulties a therapist faces under these initial circumstances: placing oneself under pressure to succeed and under the surveillance of official institutions, standing up to the continual threat of roles colliding, etc. We discuss this problem too in Sect. 4.2.

3. Finally, a third argument is that assuming responsibility for society's norms being obeyed is irreconciliable with one's identity as therapist. Certainly psychotherapy for behaviour which contravenes specific social norms is anything but simple. The problems become particularly clear when therapy not only involves actual responsibility for the wellbeing of an individual, but also forms part of a research project which produces research results and makes them available to others. It would be easy to reproach therapy for being nothing more than an *adaptation strategy* intended to enable the patient to fit in with stated norms, no matter how meaningful or senseless any one of them might be. This is a reproach which has been directed at psychotherapy in general (see the debate on criticism of psychotherapy in *Argument,* pp. 60, 71, 78, 89; in *Kursbuch,* pp. 28, 29, cited from Sigusch (1977); Sigusch (1980) has summarized and reinterpreted the discussion).

The implicit danger of passive adaptation to norms in any psychotherapy becomes particularly clear in a research project such as ours. Therapy for violation of norms always implies, explicitly or otherwise, the intention or at least the hope that in the end the norms will no longer be contravened. This generates a sense of uneasiness which can easily be backed by examples: we no longer treat homosexual patients as homosexuality among adults is no longer punishable by law in the FRG. But how would a project like this have looked 20 years ago? What might happen to the exhibitionists who constitute a large portion of our patients? If one day the relevant article is abolished from the penal code, shall we be faced with the dilemma of having treated "healthy" individuals who were only declared patients by legal clauses?

Once confronted by clinical reality the problem appears in a different light however: in a society which erects taboos, those who violate the taboos are not as a rule in a strong enough position to be able to resist them and so induce change. They are rather the people who break down under the taboos, who fail and are stranded, not only because society, with its norms and watchdogs, is stronger. A person who habitually infringes on taboos, who feels compelled to break them again and again is not going to become, as it were, automatically "healthy" once the taboos are dropped. Compulsive infringement of taboos is frequently an enactment of inner conflicts, a neurotic symptom formation accompanied by subjective distress which cannot be put down alone to suffering from the social consequences. The objection that redefining contravention of norms as an individual's intrapsychic symptom is only a more subtle kind of adaptation manoeuvre disregards the patients' real situation, or at least that of sex offenders.

No matter which direction this ideological discussion may take, an individual who compulsively infringes on norms is someone actually weighed down by a sense of hopelessness, subjective failure and suffering; the therapist must feel moved to provide help, quite independently of any ideological considerations. "It will often only be a question of not letting the patient perish and of fighting the psychical and social misery which affects him so deeply. There is then no justification for reproaching a therapist for using passive adaptation therapy. Anyone who denies the need for therapeutic work to aid adaptation from the lofty heights of theory and names no currently practicable alternatives, ignores reality and takes a cynical view of medical responsibility" (Sigusch 1980, p. 409).

1.2 The History and Development of the Research Project

Working in the Department of Sex Research makes it impossible to overlook or reconcile oneself to the dilemma that there is a lack of therapeutic concepts for patients who have developed perverse symptoms.[1] In our outpatient clinic we are confronted time and again with these problems. Another traditional focus in the department is to provide forensic reports on sexual delinquents. Given our idea of ourselves as therapists, it is very dissatisfying to be restricted to producing expertises, not only because the therapeutic recommendations which frequently thrust themselves on us are little more than theoretical wishful thinking without any chance of being implemented, but also because we are constantly confronted by relapses due to the lack of therapeutic care.

Preliminary work on the project began in 1974, initially in the form of a literature survey. We found no systematic studies we could have built on. The most we found were some approaches in behaviour therapy literature; the difficulty there however was that the concept of sexual deviancy propagated did not

[1] In this book we have used both the terms sexual deviation, sexual deviancy as well as the concept perversion, and the adjectives deviant and perverse. They are not synonyms. We use *deviancy, deviation* when outwardly *describing a behaviour* and *perversion* to characterize *intrapsychic symptom formation* from a psychodynamic angle. Sexual aggression against a woman, for example, is a deviant action, but is not necessarily a perverse symptom formation.

coincide with our theoretical position. Nonetheless, we started *pragmatically* by adopting a number of *directive methods* from behaviour therapy literature: techniques to improve self-control which were meant to help the patient master his deviant symptoms better and, in addition, some elements of assertion training to improve social skills and involving the partner in various forms of couple therapy (see Sect. 4.4 for details).

Despite all the changes in focus and method which this project has undergone and which we shall outline here, these elements always remained a part of our therapeutic procedure, although with a different emphasis. Using them did not mean however that we accepted the basic assumptions implicit in behaviour therapy concepts of treatment. Concepts such as "treatment programmes", pieced together as a mosaic of different techniques, tempt one to make the simple theoretical assumption that deviant symptoms are the expression and outcome of "behaviour deficits" or inadequate learning which have, as it were, just to be repaired so that the deviation becomes superfluous. In our view, this line of thinking is short-sighted and results in a misleading view of the problems involved.

When project funding began (1975), we had already benefitted from four years' work in an ongoing *Balint group* and had invited a female psychoanalyst to join the team at an early stage: both factors gave us access to new and important insights. It soon emerged that the behaviour therapy methods mentioned could only be applied successfully to a relatively small number of our patients and met with the more or less explicit resistance of others. During supervision of the therapies we learned that the acceptability and effectiveness of directive techniques are heavily dependent on the nature and quality of the therapeutic relationship and, furthermore, that a behaviour therapy approach to the symptom can only be properly directed if the psychodynamic background and the significance and function of the perverse symptoms in a patient's psychological equilibrium have been analysed and understood. In this context we gradually became aware of the enormous variety and complexity of the personality disorders which can lie behind perverse symptoms.

In order to deepen and systematize these insights we arranged *regular cooperation with psychoanalysts* from the Michael Balint Insitute of Psychoanalysis and Psychotherapy in Hamburg over a period of 2 years. This cooperation consisted mostly of patients, who we had examined and admitted to the therapy project, being interviewed again by a psychoanalyst. In joint case seminars the patient's problems, diagnosis and possible therapeutic approaches were discussed. The psychoanalysts also carried out a few therapies.[2] Occasionally we presented and jointly discussed our ongoing therapies.

Looking back on the initial phase of this cooperation, it seemed difficult and irksome. Given the traditionally reluctant contact between different psychotherapeutic "schools", it proved difficult to find a common level on which to

[2] These therapies are not included in our evaluation as the parallel research methods were not adopted.

communicate. Particularly our behaviourist approach and techniques met with much scepticism and were regarded merely as a kind of "anteroom exercise" before therapy proper began. A fairly long process of getting acquainted was needed until productive cooperation finally set in. We learned a great deal from this joint work:

- A deeper understanding of perverse symptoms, their roots in a personality problem and their stabilizing function for inner equilibrium.
- A more differentiated view of the therapist-patient relationship as regards phenomena known in psychoanalysis as transference and countertransference.
- A broader understanding of the therapeutic process. We have come closer to discovering why particular kinds of intervention are or are not successful at specific moments in therapy. We have gradually learnt that directive intervention, in particular, has to be seen in the context of transference and countertransference; only then can it be meaningfully implemented.

Introducing psychodynamic ideas into behaviour therapy methods is not new (see particularly Wittmann 1981; Pohlen and Wittmann 1983). This has been facilitated by developments in behaviour therapy in which the therapist-patient relationship and interaction between the two are taken into account and analysed. Using a different theoretical perspective and different terminology it is possible to take account of the phenomena termed transference, countertransference and resistance in psychoanalytic language. For this approach, other tendencies in recent behaviour therapy are also important: moving away from the classical behaviourist method, where isolating single kinds of behaviour ("symptoms") and analysing the changes brought about by conditioning factors formed the only basis for diagnosis and therapy. In this process a much needed "vertical" behaviour analysis has been introduced to complement and broaden the classical "horizontal" analysis (Grawe and Dziewas 1977). *Vertical behaviour analysis* places single kinds of behaviour in the context of overlapping, hierarchically ordered "interaction plans". By abstracting patterns from individual forms of behaviour, selective interaction and strategies for coping with life can be extrapolated. These largely correspond to defence mechanisms if they are manifested in behaviour (see p. 51). They point to the anxieties and conflicts which underlie them, not only to consciously ("cognitively") accessible emotions but also to unconscious mechanisms. Even the therapeutic relationship ("interaction") can be analysed as the interplay of "interaction plans" in an "interaction pattern" and employed therapeutically. Functional vertical behaviour analysis is an instrument which enables one to view behaviour, emotions and defence mechanisms in a dynamic context.

Our diagnostic and therapeutic approach was influenced more and more by psychodynamic thinking the further our project developed. We specifically do not regard our concept as a potpourri of behaviour therapy and psychoanalysis or a new kind of "multidimensional" approach in which elements from behaviour therapy and psychoanalysis function side by side like separate pieces in a "therapy programme" mosaic. Our view is that, at least for patients with such complex problems, psychodynamic thinking and understanding form an indispensable basis for well-placed and useful application of directive techniques. In Sect. 4.4 we describe our concept for this therapeutic procedure and how we tried to implement it.

We were encouraged in this therapeutic procedure not least by our experience in cooperating with psychoanalysts: just as a classical behaviour therapy and symptom-oriented method often does not have any effect on these patients, the psychoanalysts found in their albeit small number of therapies with these patients that the classical psychoanalytic setting was not particularly promising and that it had to be modified by a more directive and active approach, such as has been described by Fürstenau (1977) and Kernberg (1975), inter alia. The slight tendency towards a *convergence of therapeutic methods* is further evidence of the need for an interlinking of empathic, confronting, supportive and active-directive procedures with varied emphases, depending on the specific problems involved, provided this is backed up by a carefully considered therapeutic theory.

The changes in method and focus in the course of the project created special methodological problems when we came to evaluate the project. The changes which evolved during the entire procees and modified the thrust of our investigation and our objectives prevented us from applying the classical model of psychotherapy research: the pre-post design. We describe how we dealt with these methodological problems, and how we tried to resolve them, in Sect. 3.1.

1.3 Survey of Literature

1.3.1 Behaviour Therapy for Sexual Deviancy

The literature on treatment of sexual deviancy has paid little attention to more recent developments in behaviour therapy, particulary regarding the relevance of the therapeutic relationship and the understanding of a symptom in the context of a patient's history. In this respect, behaviour therapy has still to catch up on lost ground in its own development. It is dominated by *one-dimensional therapy studies,* particularly single case studies, in which deviant behaviour is treated in isolation using separate behaviour therapy techniques. Most of the investigations focus pragmatically on therapy methods or examine the value of psychophysiological methods of assessment for diagnosis and evaluation of changes. Aetilogical aspects and symptom interpretation are for the most part ignored and are rarely considered when choosing a therapeutic strategy. The dissatisfaction with this isolation of symptoms recently led to the development of a *multimodal approach* in which several "areas of disturbance" are examined and treated with the appropriate techniques.

1.3.1.1 Aetiological Models in Learning Theory

Yates' (1970) observation that behaviour therapists show little interest in formulating theories on the genesis and reinforcement of sexually deviant behaviour is still true today. Neither a concept of sexuality in general nor an elaborated theory on the genesis of sexual deviancy is available. So far only vague attempts have been made which are at best fragments of a theory.

McGuire et al. (1977) developed an approach oriented on the models of classical and operant conditioning. They assume that every environmental stimulus may acquire sexual significance. The determining factor in the evolution of sexual deviation is allegedly the first time a neutral stimulus (e.g. a piece of underwear for a future underwear fetishist or a punishment scene for a future sadomasochist) coincides with sexual arousal, so that both stimuli become linked. Masturbation and phantasies are important in maintaining this combination as, on the one hand, they satisfy sexual desire and, on the other, can provide protection from fears of failure with the opposite sex (Metzner 1963). Similar assumptions formed the basis of experiments by Rachman (1966) and Rachman and Hodgson (1969) who conditioned an artificial, temporary "fetishism". On the basis of the social learning model (Bandura and Walters 1963), Bandura (1969) developed the hypothesis that deviant sexual behaviour is also acquired and indirectly reinforced through behaviour models.

1.3.1.2 Behaviour Therapy Techniques

The most frequently employed behaviour therapy techniques focus on the deviant sexual symptom itself. The early fundamental concept behind behaviour therapy, i.e. interpreting the symptom as an isolated or at least separable disturbance which can be directly treated, has been favoured for a long time - probably inspired by the provocative, norm-breaking dimensions of the symptom. Of these *symptom-focussed intervention techniques* aversive methods have been clearly preferred to nonaversive ones for getting rid of the symptom. *Methods not exclusively focussed on the symptom* try to remove "behaviour deficits" and thereby make the deviant symptom superfluous.

Symptom-Focussed Methods

Aversive Conditioning. A large number of techniques have been developed under the label "aversive conditioning"; their aim is to suppress sexual arousability caused by deviant stimuli by using aversive stimuli. The idea is to associate deviant stimuli with aversive stimuli in order to change the deviant stimuli to conditioned aversive stimuli. After attempts with chemical aversion stimuli failed (e.g. Davis and Morgenstern 1960; Cooper 1963) owing to their side effects (Rachman and Teasdale 1969), electric shock techniques were gradually elaborated: variation of the shock type, strength, duration, place and kind of application. Such forms of avoidance and escape learning go beyond mere punishment: a lack of shock or termination of shocks is coupled with nondeviant stimuli. The aim was for nondeviant stimuli to acquire a positive significance. The following authors carried out the various kinds of "aversive conditioning", sometimes combined with other methods: Raymond (1956, 1969), Fookes (1969), Blakemoore et al. (1963), Thorpe et al. (1964), Clark (1965), Marks et al. (1965), Marks and Gelder (1967), Bond and Evans (1967), Evans (1967,1968, 1970), Feldmann et al. (1968), Abel et al. (1970), Marshall 1971, 1973, 1974, Gaupp et al. (1971), McCulloch et al. (1971), Rosenthal (1973), Marshall and McKnight (1975), Mathis (1975), Miller and Haney (1976), Pinard and Lamontagne (1976), Wickramasekera (1977), Rhodes and Levinson (1977), Schmieschek (1977), Wijesinghe (1977), Dummer and Burian (1978), Nolan and Sandman (1978), Josiassen et al. (1980).

Aversive conditioning was soon questioned: its efficacy has been doubted (for example, by Bandura 1962; Powell and Azrin 1968; Barlow 1973). It has been rejected on moral grounds (e.g. by Appel 1964) and criticized for such serious long-term effects as aggression, depression, psychosomatic disorders (e.g. Appel 1964; Cooper 1963).

Shame Aversion Therapy. Shame aversion therapy (Serber 1970) was employed on patients with exhibitionist symptoms (Reitz and Keil 1971; Serber 1972; Stevenson and Jones 1972; Boudwyns et al. 1975; Mathis 1975; Wickramasekera 1977; Jones and Frei 1977; Wardlaw and Miller 1978). The patients were asked to expose themselves in front of women who were instructed to mock at them. The mockery was used as an aversive stimulus.

Covert Sensitization. Covert sensitization is a cognitive method of aversive symptom control. An imagined situation is used as an aversive stimulus: the patient is instructed to imagine a situation in which deviant acts frequently take place and to link it to repellent images. The aversive thoughts are intended to become a reflex which interrupts the chain of behaviour and eliminates arousability by deviant stimuli. Apart from aversive conditioning, this is the most frequently mentioned technique and is often combined with other methods (Kolvin 1967; Davison 1968; Barlow et al. 1969; Gershman 1970; Cautela and Wisocki 1971; Burdick 1972; Glick 1972; Callahan and Leitenberg 1973; Fensterheim 1974; Harbert et al. 1974; Mathis 1975; McKay 1976; Brownell and Barlow 1976; Hughes 1977; Boudreau et al. 1978; Hayes et al. 1978; Kurlychek 1978; Alford et al. 1980; Maletzky 1974, 1977, 1980).

Negative Exercise. Occasionally the negative exercise method has been employed, also referred to as the "satiation" method or "induced boredom" (Marshall and Lippens 1977; Marshall 1979; Gretenkord 1981). Given the importance of masturbation phantasies in sustaining deviant behaviour (McGuire et al. 1977), patients were asked to masturbate continuously for a long period, even beyond ejaculation, using deviant phantasies. To check on him the patient was, for example, observed behind a one-way mirror and had to speak his phantasies out loud. It was expected that the patient would in the end literally lose any desire.

Symptom Control Using Biofeedback. Rosen and Kopel (1977) used biofeedback techniques to aid deliberate control of sexual arousability through deviant stimuli; other authors have used it in combination with other methods (Laws 1980; Quinsey et al. 1980; Gretenkord 1981).

Self-management Methods. Self-management methods do not aim at suppressing arousability by sexual stimuli, but at deliberately preventing deviant behaviour. Self-management methods have acquired some significance in behaviour therapy (see Kanfer 1977; Reinecker 1978), but only play a minor role in the treatment of sexually deviant behaviour (Bancroft 1974, 1983; Rooth and Marks 1974; Snaith and Collins 1981).

Methods not Exclusively Focussed on the Symptom

Conditioning Sexual Arousability with Nondeviant Stimuli. A summary of this method is to be found in Abel et al. (1974). Based on the ideas of McGuire et al. (1977) on the role of masturbation phantasies, Marquis (1970) developed the method of orgasmic reconditioning using Davison's (1968) method: the patient is asked to switch just before orgasm to nondeviant images which can still arouse him. The procedure of switching thoughts is introduced earlier each time until deviant phantasies can eventually be dispensed with. This method was used, sometimes combined with others, by the following authors: Marshall (1973, 1974, 1979), Herman et al. (1974), Conrad and Wince (1976), Miller and Haney (1976), Beech et al. (1971), Boudreau et al. (1978), Van Deventer and Laws (1978), Kremsdorf et al. (1980), Lande (1980), Foot and Laws (1981).

Systematic Desensitization of Social and Sexual Anxieties and Increasing Social Skills. The use of systematic desensitization for patients with sexually deviant symptoms is based on the assumption that social and sexual anxieties are mitigated by deviant acts. Techniques for increasing social skills aim more at reducing behaviour deficits. These methods were often used in a highly mechanical fashion; occasionally they were linked to a more differentiated view of the underlying problem (Wolpe 1958; Stevenson and Wolpe 1960; Dengrove 1967; Marshall 1971; Serber 1972; Edwards 1972; Kohlenberg 1974; Miller and Haney 1976; Schmiescheck 1977; Seiderer-Hartig 1977; Bond and Hutchinson 1964; Boudreau et al. 1978; Keltner et al. 1978; Crawford and Allen 1979; Langevin et al. 1979; Josiassen et al. 1980).

Sex Therapy and Couple Therapy. Based on the idea that the need for deviant sexuality loses its significance if "normal sexuality" in a "normal" partnership is satisfying, the authors carried out sex therapy, usually as an additional technique (sometimes with so-called surrogate partners) and couple therapies (Cooper 1963; Kohlenberg 1974; Bancroft 1974, 1983; Mathis 1975; Rosen and Kopel 1977; Abel et al. 1978; Groth 1979).

1.3.1.3 Multidimensional and Theory-Based Approaches in Behaviour Therapy

From the mid-1970s on some authors turned away from a focus on isolated aspects of disorders, particularly deviant arousability (Barlow 1974; Bancroft 1974, 1983; Barlow and Abel 1976; Abel et al. 1978; Crawford 1979). They emphasized the variety of personality problems and demanded a more individual therapeutic procedure. In these pragmatic, multidimensional approaches (Lazarus 1967, 1976) the authors group the various areas of disturbance and therapy approaches as follows: deviant and nondeviant sexual arousability, sexual and social anxieties, ability to relate to others and social skills, self-image and gender role identity. The therapy methods outlined above, in addition to sex education and instruction, were assigned to these areas (Mathis 1975; Miller and Haney 1976; Boudreau et al. 1978; Gretenkord 1981). The basic idea of a broad, pragmatic approach is implemented in a large number of intra- and extramural treatment programmes for sexual delinquents (see the survey by Brecher 1978), which cannot however be ascribed to any particular psychotherapeutic orientation.

Even if the multidimensional approaches do broaden perception and procedure and offer a chance of patient-oriented therapy planning, they still remain fixed on the phenomenological level of the patient's pathology. Choosing a therapy focus or method is not the result of reflecting on a theory, but rather is oriented on the availability of specific methods and programmes.

Schwartz and Masters (1983) made more use of theory and defined sexual deviance as a disturbance in establishing intimate relationships - as did Ploog et al. (1982) who attempted to reconstruct the development of sexual deviancy from the patient's history of experience and learning. They tried to use behaviour therapy interventions, which they saw from a psychodynamic angle.

1.3.1.4 Criticism of Orthodox Behaviour Therapy

There is a lack of an elaborated learning theory on sexual deviations as a basis and background for therapeutic practice. The theories mentioned above which trace the origins of sexual deviation back to a (coincidental) coupling of sexual arousal with neutral stimuli are too simple. The explanation is unconvincing since it has to recourse to coincidence (the chance linking of stimulus and reaction). Important life experiences are easily disregarded when applying concepts from learning theory. Ploog et al. (1982), for example, attempted to analyse the development and maintenance of a patient's aggressive sexual acts against children, using learning theory concepts. They found that the most important aspects of development could not be traced. The "anaemic" impression made by the terms used is especially evident in the reduction of sexuality to "sexual arousability" and its physiological aspects which can then of course be measured using advanced technology. This theoretical approach reaches its climax in the definition of sexual deviation as "deviant sexual arousability" in the *Diagnostic Statistical Manual of the American Psychiatry Association* (according to Crawford 1979).

The lack of aetiological explanations obstructs any understanding of the function of deviant sexuality in maintaining the person's psychological equilibrium. It is not enough to interpret deviant sexual symptoms just as avoidance and substitute behaviour stemming from fears of failure in heterosexual situations.

This blindness to the meaning and function of deviant symptoms handicaps the definition of appropriate therapy goals. The theoretical notion of deviant sexual arousability as an entity in itself justifies using aversive methods to remove the symptoms, regardless of whether this might eventually destabilize the patient. Combining this method with others for developing alternative behaviour does not remove this danger, as it focusses on the phenomenology of patients' anxieties and "deficits", but not on understanding these anxieties.

The danger is that therapeutic methods are used arbitrarily. The conclusion to be drawn from the investigations mentioned which experiment with the efficacy of intervention techniques is rather meagre: each method was said to be both successful and unsuccessful in therapy. There are also methodological reasons for this. Single case studies can only demonstrate whether a therapy, in which a particular technique was used, was successful or not. The reasons for success or failure remain unclear. Systematic investigations only check on the variables which are easiest to get hold of experimentally; whether these variables are the most essential ones remains doubtful. It seems that a combination of several methods has more chance of success than only one method. Apart from this, there are no other reliable conclusions to be drawn from these investigations.

The tendency to search for greater technical sophistication in therapeutic procedure shows that the therapeutic relationship and the interaction process betweeen patient and therapist are widely ignored. This does not of course mean that the therapist-patient relationship is unlikely ever to be a decisive factor in this kind of therapy. For example: aversion techniques used as a vehicle for socially sanctioned counteraggression, which can moreover link up with the patient's need to be punished, divide the power between therapist and patient very unevenly and identify the therapist with a punitive authority. Shame aversion therapy works by depreciating and degrading the patient; covert sensitisation appeals to the patient's desire to be punished and his feelings of guilt; biofeedback and orgasmic reconditioning methods force the patient to disclose highly intimate thoughts, etc. The success or failure of these forms of therapy clearly depends more on the patient's reaction to the kind of therapeutic relationship than on the quality of the method. This criticism applies equally to therapy using non-punitive techniques. As long as the perspective fails to encompass two pivotal dimensions - analysis of the therapeutic relationship and a broader understanding of the context - the course of therapy remains random and arbitrary, and the therapeutic potential of (nonpunitive) behaviour therapy methods cannot be made use of. To this extent we concur with more recent developments in behaviour therapy (for example, Pohlen and Wittmann 1983).

1.3.2 Psychoanalytic Literature on the Treatment of Sexual Delinquents

We dispense with a complete, synoptic review of psychoanalytic literature on perversions here. In Sects. 3.2 and 3.3 we discuss in detail the aspects of psychoanalytic theory and its implications for therapy which are relevant to our inquiry and understanding. The large number of case studies in psychoanalytic perversion research (for example: Eissler 1958; Robertiello 1971; Stolorow and Grand 1973; Goldberg 1975; Haag 1980) is of little help for our investigation. As a rule they discuss highly selected patients with characteristics that differ fundamentally from those of our patients; they were, moreover, in most cases treated for their own (inner) problems with their perversion and not for delinquent behaviour.

Essentially, we found eight studies which explicitly discussed *therapy for sexual delinquents* and not just single case description.

Stürüp (1963) and Sachs (1965) reported on therapy for sexual delinquents assigned to a special institution in Herstedvester, Denmark. The reports are based on a large number of patients (Stürüp: 81, Sachs: 78). Type and duration of psychotherapy are not described in detail. Goudsmit and Reicher (1980) also report on years of *intramural* psychotherapy for delinquents in the Van Mesdag Clinic in Groningen, Holland, some of whom were sexual delinquents. Jessen (1969) reports on intramural treatment results in the Van der Hoeven Clinic in Utrecht, Holland.

This leaves four studies which analysed *outpatient* treatment of sexual delinquents more systematically - i.e. they resemble more closely our overall framework. Conn (1949) treated 23 patients accused of different offences using analytic short-term therapy. Duration of treatment was between 6 months and 5 years. Follow-up reports are available; 19 therapies were considered successful.

Bräutigam (1966) reports on the treatment of 12 sex offenders given psychoanalytically oriented, short-term therapy. Bräutigam used Goudsmit's three-phase model: the "contact treatment" phase is followed by a phase of "ego reinforcement", followed by psychoanalytic therapy itself. Of these, 10 therapies were conducted successfully ("improved"), follow-ups are only partially available.

Hackett (1971) reports on outpatient psychotherapeutic treatment of 37 exhibitionists. After treatment lasting between 6 months and 14 years 33 therapies were successful; this was confirmed by follow-ups.

Petri (1980) carried out psychoanalytic short-term therapy with 20 patients with differing symptoms, combining it with anti-androgen treatment. Therapy was successful in 11 patients, confirmed in follow-ups.

An important aspect of these investigations is that, after making a critical and realistic assessment, they all conclude that psychotherapy has a good effect on these patients. They demonstrate, above all, that prejudices against an apparent lack of distress or motivation for therapy are unjustified. Nevertheless this approach has not been followed up.

2 Description of the Research Project

2.1 Sample Selection

Between 1975 and 1980 a total of 169 patients were indicated for psychotherapeutic treatment. We excluded those patients:

- Who were psychotic or were seriously addicted
- Whose ability to communicate verbally was insufficient due to mental deficiency or brain damage
- Who were in prison or committed to psychiatric hospitals
- Who had been sentenced and were expected to go to prison during or shortly after therapy

Patients who only showed a minimal willingness to cooperate in therapy were deliberately not excluded. We wanted to resist the temptation of applying this common selection criterion, which relativizes the significance of success rates in most investigations, for the following reasons: first, assessment of therapy motivation is subjective and also influenced by sympathy/antipathy; second, this assessment depends on the extent to which the investigator makes contact with the patient and develops empathy for his dilemma. After all, a patient who is liable to be prosecuted faces a situation with his therapist which cannot be compared with that of a patient in a traditional psychotherapy setting. The humiliation of his offence, moral self-condemnation, his suspicion of any possible connection to the legal authorities in cases where the court has ordered treatment, etc., can seriously influence a patient's willingness to display any personal interest in therapy. Moreover, many of these patients have little idea what psychotherapy is and do not know what to expect. We assumed that awakening or strengthening their own interest in themselves might in itself be an important achievement in therapeutic work (see Sect. 4.2).

The indication criteria were deliberately kept formal as we wanted to collect *a broad range* of experience and avoid screening out too many patients from the start by applying too narrow criteria, e.g. those involving "motivation" and "distress". We wanted to find a realistic answer to the question which patients from the group of nonimprisoned sex offenders were accessible to psychotherapeutic treatment.

Of the 169 patients 49 (29%) did not embark on therapy ("waiting-list dropouts"). Of the patients who were still on the waiting list at the end of the project, 34 were assigned to therapists outside our institute. In the following we ar referring to a *therapy sample of n = 86.*

Of these 86 patients, 22 or about one quarter broke off therapy prematurel in the view of the therapists. Our decision to nonetheless include these *dropou* in our sample was based on the following considerations: criteria definin when therapy has been concluded or discontinued vary greatly; they depen on the therapeutic concept and the therapist's subjective notions of success an failure which by no means always coincide with the patient's expectations an ideas. The decisive criterion for inclusion in the sample was whether any thera py had taken place at all, even if only very briefly, as in some cases. Exclusio of the therapy dropouts would have improved our success rate, but would hav led to an unrealistic assessment of the potential of outpatient psychotherapeu tic treatment for this patient group: we would have bracketed out a group c patients who benefit less from therapy.

2.2 Design

Patients were seen in an *initial interview* by a consultant who did not conduct therapy later an was meant to act later as an independent assessor of therapy outcome. Faced with large gap in our data due to fluctuation in personnel, we had to relinquish this plan. Data were gathere on the patient's biography, psychosexual development and current social and psychologic situation in the form of a nonstandardized, carefully documented initial interview and a stan dard evaluation of the current acuteness of the deviant symptom.

A *second interview,* this time by the therapist, took place at the *start of therapy* after a waitin period (on average 9 months) using the same methods. The standardized data from the two in terviews form the basis for the control group.

The *therapies* were documented as the therapists chose; therapy planning and implementa tion were discussed in regular team meetings and supervised in a Balint group.

At the end of therapy, the therapist wrote a detailed final report. The *first follow-up* at th end of therapy was conducted both by the therapist and the first consultant using the abov methods and, additionally, a standardized method for recording modifications (overall asses ment of changes in the patient's psychological, social and sexual problems).

The *second and third follow-ups* were conducted in the same manner 1 and 3 years later. N further follow-up has taken place since. The follow-up period covered is however longer fo those patients who got in touch with us again of their own accord.

The evaluation of the initially standardized data collected is only one of the methodologic aspects of our investigation. More important when documenting the patients' intrapsych problems and the therapeutic process was subsequently standardizing the unstructured docu ments (notes, reports, expertises) using a rating method which we outline in Sect. 3.1.

Gathering data proved more difficult than we had initially suspected. The relatively hig loss of data reflects above all the patients' motivation problems, their suspicion of any kind o documentation and attempts to check on them. This explains why our data reveal some gap not only in the follow-ups but also in the initial examinations. All in all, the actual sample si varies slightly from variable to variable. There are particularly large gaps in the test data.

2.3 Data Evaluation

The relative frequency figures given for each individual variable always refer to the actual sample size.

For statistical analysis of *two variables* the following methods were used:

- Nominal and ordinal scale data: the chi-square test for independent samples and/or the Fisher exact probability test and the contingency coefficient C
- Nominal scale data with repeated measurement: the sign test
- Nominal or ordinal scale data and at least interval-scale data: the t-test and a one-way analysis of variance
- Interval-scale data with repeated measurements; t-test for dependent samples

Cluster and factor analysis was used for the statistical analysis of *several variables*.

2.4 Waiting-List Dropouts

Waiting-list dropouts (n = 49) were compared with the therapy sample (n = 86) using variables from the initial interview and the test data. There are only a few significant differences between the two samples, most of which are not particularly pronounced (C = between 0.20 and 0.37). Waiting-list dropouts are on average slightly younger. Most of the significant differences involve variables in sexual deviancy: it is less insistent in waiting-list dropouts, fewer of these patients have been previously convicted for sex offences and, if not self-motivated, they are more frequently under court order. Moreover, the decision to accept or reject therapy seems to depend more on the patients' current social situation and on coincidence than on their psychodynamic structure or problem.

2.5 Description of Therapy Sample According to External Criteria

Sexual Deviancy and Criminality

Table 1 lists the type of offence.

Table 1. Type of sexual offence

	Therapy n	sample %	Prosecuted sexual offences in the FRG, 1980 (quoted from Federal Bureau of Statistics) %
Indecent exposure to women	25	29	20
Indecent exposure to children	21	24	
Sexual acts against children	23	27	42
Violent sexual acts against women	11	13	36
Other (voyeurism, telephone harassment, fetishism)	6	7	2
Total	86	100	100

Nonviolent sexual offences are clearly over-represented in our sample; none theless, a quarter of our patients acted violently, 8% excessively so. This selec tion can easily be explained. Violent sexual offences as a rule lead to more se vere sentences and usually mean imprisonment or compulsory commitment For these reasons alone, such patients are frequently not offered the opportuni ty to undergo outpatient psychotherapy. Furthermore, the patients' psychologi cal structure plays a certain role. A comparison of violent and nonviolent se: offenders (see Schorsch 1971) shows that nonviolent offenders are frequentl better integrated socially. Isolated aberrant behaviour of a sexual kind i: accordingly more often defined as a psychological problem or illness by pa tients, and by courts and experts, and is seen as an indication for psychother apy. Moreover, the next step for most people is to judge distinctly injurious be haviour along moral lines, while it is more difficult to understand it as : psychological problem troubling the offender.

Independently of the type of offence, most of the patients' (three quarters deviant behaviour followed a firmly established conflict-solving pattern, some times becoming more severe (Table 2).

Table 2. Intensity of sexual deviancy

	n	%
Unique/sporadic, no firmly established deviancy	20	23
Frequent occurrence; firmly established deviancy, no increase in severity	48	56
Increasing severity	18	21
Total	86	100

The *acuteness of the deviancy* in terms of the frequency of phantasies and enactments varie considerably but is generally relatively strong: about two thirds of the patients report very fre quent deviant wishes, sometimes several a day; about one third enact the symptom at leas once a month. One fifth experienced no deviant wishes at the start of therapy. The *duration* (*symptoms* tended to be long-standing: almost three quarters had had the symptom for mor than 5 years, almost half for more than 10 years. Three quarters of the patients had already be come aware of their symptom in adolescence; besides these, a small group was identifie whose symptom only emerged in their forties.

A large number of the patients (two thirds) had been *previously convicted* for sexual ol fences, a quarter for nonsexual offences. One third had already been imprisoned or, less ofter committed to psychiatric treatment.

About half of the patients started therapy because they had been put under pressure by *court order* or while prosecution was pending. Some had been told about the opportunity t undergo therapy by the police without having been prosecuted. Immediately after imprisor ment or commitment 12 patients began therapy. All of these variables are statistically indeper dent of the type of offence.

Social and Biographical Data

Patient *age* was between 16 and 54 years (mean: 33 years). The great majority (three quarters) was aged between their early twenties and late thirties.

A rough distribution of *social status* is shown in Table 3.

There was no significant difference between our patients and the general population. The distinctly lower social status of sexual offenders recorded in criminal statistics is not evident in this therapy sample. On the other hand, as the social status of our patients is distinctly lower than is usual for psychotherapy patients, this selection criterion has little effect here.

Table 3. Social status

	Therapy sample %	General population (according to Janowitz 1958) %
Upper/upper middle class	2	5
Lower middle class	34	38
Upper working class	24	13
Lower working class	34	39
Unclassifiable	6	5
Total	100	100

Distribution of *school education* presents a similar picture: Only a small fraction (11%) had no secondary school certificate, most (two thirds) had this certificate and about one fifth had had further school education.

When more differentiated variables are included, many patients showed signs of *social destabilization*: some of the patients showed abnormalities in variables reflecting adverse conditions during socialization. About one fifth of the patients were born *illegitimately*; this is more than in the national population (5%-12%, Federal statistics 1963). Two fifths of the patients had lived away from home or in an incomplete family, at least for a period, and 14% of the patients for longer periods in *homes*. Just under half had suffered from *behavioural disorders* such as bed-wetting, stuttering, running away, theft during childhood. About two fifths had an *unstable employment history*, were often unemployed and frequently changed jobs; about one fifth was currently unemployed. About two fifths had no *steady partner* and as a rule were socially isolated. The other patients, too, were restricted to contact with their partner or, less often, their family. An overall *assessment of their social situation* showed that about half were only partially integrated socially, about one third clearly lived on the fringe of society. Partnerships were generally unstable or handicapped by serious conflicts.

Attitudes to Sex

Almost half the patients had a distinctly *bashful* or *embarrassed attitude* toward sex. More than two fifths had hardly any or had no sexual experience with a partner. Two fifths had pronounced *fear of failure*, one fifth *fear of sexual dysfunction*. Estimates by Arentewicz and Schmidt (1983) produced distinctly lower values for the general population. For about half the patients sexuality had an exaggerated, sometimes extreme importance; in about three quarters of the patients this was, however, coupled with an almost total absence of close relationships.

Clinical Symptoms

About two thirds of the patients showed other symptoms: *alcohol and drug addiction* (two fifths), though the role played by medication was small and that of hard drugs almost negligible; a *depressive syndrome*, including a tendency towards suicide, was observed in one half and *psychosomatic symptoms* in one third. If one also counts *criminality* as a symptom, then only about one fifth of patients had no symptoms apart from their sexual deviancy.

Here too there proved to be a concentration on one group of patients: one half of the symptoms accumulated around one third of the patients, and four fifths of symptoms around about one half of the patients.

3 Diagnosis: The Structure and Psychodynamics of Patients' Inner Problems

3.1 Research Strategy and Problems of Method

3.1.1 Research Strategy

The demographic and standardized data recorded are external data and give us little help in understanding the patients' inner dynamics. The patient's history is the best source for a clear analysis and description of his conflicts and structure, of the meaning and significance of his symptoms. With all our information on 86 mostly well documented and analysed cases we hoped to find a *broad empirical basis* - regarding not only the heterogeneity of the structures and problems involved, but also the great variety of possible psychodynamic ramifications of a perverse symptom. An appropriate method had to be found to do this.

The literature on the psychodynamic diagnosis of sexual perversions can be separated roughly into two groups: first, *theoretical studies* which discuss metapsychological aspects (recently, for example, Morgenthaler 1974, 1984; Stoller 1975; Khan 1979), often enriched and illustrated by one or two patient histories which become self-evident through the selection process and, second, *single case studies* which are discussed in connection with certain theoretical stances.

We had the choice between two methods of approach:

1. Describing and *stringing together numerous case examples*. The advantage of this approach lies in its clarity: by reading such a broad variety of cases general structures and set patterns can become apparent.

2. Methodical *distillation of general structures and set patterns*. This method has the disadvantage of loss in clarity as it has to function on a more abstract level. Above all, it involves breaking down a specific, clear gestalt (history, structure, problems of a patient and the interwoven perverse symptom) into separate parts which are handled one at a time, despite the fact that the separation or isolation of an interwoven component part is artificial.

It seemed to us sensible and obvious to combine and interlock the two approaches. When isolating and discussing separate aspects below - for instance: the different aspects of the meaning of the symptom, various personality problem areas, defence mechanisms and coping strategies - we shall illustrate them with case examples. Our use of case histories here fulfills a double function: first, it is meant to document concrete evidence of the isolated aspect and describe it lucidly. Second, the patient's history is used to show that each aspect is a component part of a whole, thereby relating it again to the gestalt as a whole. Accordingly, case histories take up a relatively large space, especially as we document the history, diagnosis assessment, therapy progress and outcome for each of the 18 examples. We have dispensed with sketching vignettes or partial aspects when giving examples as they can all too easily seem to be tailored to illustrate only one particular aspect.

3.1.2 Method

In Sect. 1.2 we described how the process of developing the research project brought about changes which affected both our diagnostic perspective and, above all, our therapeutic method. The changes which took place forced us to recognize, among other things, that these patients needed a particularly flexible and individual therapeutic approach, if any therapeutic process at all was to be initiated and to avoid the patient having to reject what was essentially a helpful opportunity. The common method in therapy research of exclusive *orientation on research outcome* along the lines of a *pre-post design* therefore proved inappropriate for our research project. Limiting ourselves to simply evaluating therapy outcome would have meant bypassing the essential focus of this research project and ignoring one of our main interests: the development, description and explanation of the therapeutic procedure and process.

Furthermore the ongoing modifications to the project showed that the categories used for diagnostic classification and for the therapeutic process, which we considered essential, could only be the *result* of our research. Consequently *parallel process research with preset categories* was rejected as unsuitable.

In order to arrive at more generally applicable theses and results than could be achieved by merely stringing together case histories, we searched for a methodological compromise and took a *hermeneutical approach,* choosing a *standardized evaluation of freely documented information by a rating group.* Our method was as follows: the rating group consisted of the five authors (three clinical psychologists, a psychoanalyst and a psychiatrist) of whom, however, only one or two had seen the patient involved. The rating of each patient was made on the evidence of all the documented material available on him.

Our procedure consisted of *six consecutive steps*:

First Step: Working Out the Main Themes

The rating group had cooperated closely over the past few years in team discussions and supervision and was therefore familiar with the subject matter. Using our joint experience, we analysed which themes and areas could be relevant for the diagnostic classification of a patient and an evaluation of the therapeutic process. The first task was to find rough headings to help orientation. We agreed on the following aspects:

For the *diagnostic classification* we chose the following themes:

Meaning and Significance of Perverse Symptoms: in supervision we had realized that this aspect was of crucial importance. The various facets of personality and its specific disorders are concentrated in the symptom and take shape as a gestalt. Understanding the symptom is, as it were, the key to each patient's problems. Moreover, we had also discovered that continually recurring, typical nonperverse problems are reflected in the symptom. This led us to outline

Typical Problem Areas: we selected four themes or aspects which are repeatedly cited in perversion literature: the *masculinity problem* and male identity, the *problem of aggression*, self-image and *experience of self*, and *problems with relationships*. For reasons of clarity one cannot avoid discussing these problem areas one after another. We are, however, aware that they are merely individual aspects of the whole, that there are no clear-cut boundaries between them, that one aspect develops out of another and that the structure of each patient is different and complex.

The typical problem areas are linked to *typical coping strategies*. In using this concept we are following a trend in contemporary behaviour therapy (Grawe and Dziewas 1977; Wittmann 1981) to adopt concepts such as interaction plans and life strategies; our definition is, however, less strict. The concept characterizes basic behaviour patterns typical of a personality and constantly recurring throughout life. In psychodynamic literature coping strategies correspond closest to defence mechanisms, i.e. the way in which defence mechanisms are reflected in behaviour (see Sect. 3.5). The typical problem areas named are manifested in the coping strategies; the coping strategies are an attempt to compensate these problems.

We settled on the following headings for documenting and *assessing the therapy process*:

- Problems of *motivation* and *distress*
- Kind, quality of and changes within the *patient-therapist relationship*
- Kind and assessment of *therapeutic procedure*
- *Results of therapy, therapy assessment*
- Appraisal of condition at *follow-up*

Second Step: Nonstandardized Evaluation of 32 Patient Histories Using These Headings

First of all we made a random selection of 32 patient histories. Each of the five raters independently assessed each of these patients using the rough headings described above. For example: what function can the sexual symptom have for this patient, which problems does it manifest, what typical coping strategies are identifiable, what special qualities are there in the therapeutic relationship, how is therapy proceeding, and so on.

Third Step: Working Towards Agreement on a Joint Assessment

In joint discussions the rating group came to a consensus on how the patients rated under the various headings. The aim was to work towards a kind of gestalt of the patient and the therapeutic process.

Fourth Step: Inductive Elaboration of Categories for a Standardized Category System

The outcome of the joint assessment formed the basis for evolving a system of categories *inductively*. For example, we listed all the meanings which had been named under the heading "the significance of the perverse symptom", extracted those which occurred more frequently and constructed categories from them. We handled all the thematic areas above in the same way. These categories are nominally or ordinally scaled using two to a maximum of five, as a rule three, gradations.

Fifth Step: Assessment of the 86 Patients Using the Standardized Category System

After testing the category system on a few patients, each of the five raters independently used this system to assess all 86 patients.

Sixth Step: Finding a Consensus on Assessment with the Category System.

In the last step we worked towards a group consensus on a joint rating. We decided against arithmetical methods of computing a final assessment; instead we agreed on the discussion and consensus method because this produces more reliable and valid results within a balanced rater group familiar with the subject matter.[1]

We believe that sufficiently objective, reliable and valid data were gathered using this exhaustive procedure. We are quite aware one can object to our method on the grounds that the rater group cannot be completely impartial and that, furthermore, retrospective process analysis always involves simplification loss of information and some distortion.

The results of the consensus ratings were included in the statistical analysis The statistical methods used are summarized in Sect. 2.3. Special problems of method are discussed again wherever the outcome of special procedures is presented.

In concluding our methodological outline, there is one common objection to consider: our project is an attempt to combine an approach involving psychodynamic categories with statistical methods. It is rather unusual to combine

[1] To assess whether agreement among the 5 raters was adequate for discussing and achieving a consensus we calculated rater agreement using Ebel (Guilford 1954). The values lay between 0.32 and 0.91 with a mean of 0.63. Agreement varied considerably among variables but was generally adequate.

these two methods and similar research initiatives are rare (for example, Dahl 1972; Thomä and Kächele 1973; Meyer 1981; Stuhr 1984).

The view that the more hermeneutical, historical approach in psychoanalysis is incompatible with statistical thinking and methods is definitely incorrect and merely reflects a lack of reciprocal knowledge between the two fields. The objection that using statistical methods within psychodynamic theory can only reproduce, but not test psychodynamic results is as obvious as it is banal since methodology can only be used as an aid within theory. Statistics which employ, for example, only hard facts imply a theoretical position in which, in the vein of crude positivism, only a reality quite free of subjectivity is at all significant. The limitation of our results consists in the fact that the conclusions drawn can apply only to the theory we used. Our results should be seen in the light of this natural limitation.

3.2 The Meaning and Function of Perverse Symptoms

3.2.1 Theoretical and Clinical Aspects

3.2.1.1 Our Theoretical Position

Since a psychodynamic understanding of perverse symptoms is fundamentally important in diagnosis, therapy and prognosis, we open this section with a discussion of this approach. As with neurotic or psychosomatic illnesses, meaningful statements about therapy are only feasible if the symptoms are viewed within the context of the entire personality. We do not intend to discuss here the complex psychoanalytic theories of sexual perversion, their historical development and modification, and refer the reader to the survey by Becker and Schorsch (1980).

We start out from the general theoretical assumption that a sexual perversion, perverse phantasies and the perverse impulse are compensatory in character and should be seen as an attempt to heal wounds. Acting out the perversion has, at least temporarily, a calming and stabilizing effect on the person's psychological equilibrium. A perverse symptom can have very different determinants and obeys the "principle of multiple function" (Wälder 1936). In perverse enactments we get a glimpse of early conflicts which influenced decisive relationships; the perverse symptoms represent complexly coded attempts at resolving these conflicts. The idea of repairing or making up for something is therefore the key to understanding the symptom. There are various basic themes and anxieties which can be expressed in perverse symptoms, for instance: the feeling that damaged male identity has been momentarily restored; a triumphant sense of being potent and powerful which temporarily compensates for otherwise feeling helpless and insignificant; the search for admiration, intimacy, warmth, a feeling of security, care, comfort, for complete symbiosis, evident in some pedophile relationships; re-experiencing infantile omnipotence; defence against anxieties such as being emasculated, devoured and annihilated by a woman; phantasies of having a person all to oneself, or of dominating someone to alleviate fears of being abandoned, etc. The priority in clinical work is to select from among these "multiple functions" those which have "motivational priority" (Stolorow 1979). They vary in each patient and have important implications for the therapeutic concept.

The specific element in perverse symptom formation is *the defence mechanism sexualization* . In a person's life sexual experiences can have a stabilizing function; they can convey consolation, confidence and pride, can appease anxieties and fulfill a variety of needs. *Excessive sexualization,* however, even in genital sexuality which seems outwardly normal (as in "Don Juanism"), is always also an indication that powerful anxieties are being warded off. Patients who develop *perverse symptoms* cannot make use of "normal" sexual contacts as a stabilizing factor since for them mature genital sexuality is linked with anxiety (see Mentzos 1982). In the early days of psychoanalytic research, perversion formation was thought to be contraphobic, a strategy for coping with castration anxieties within the oedipal conflict (Fenichel 1932). A further differentiation of psychoanalytic concepts has helped to develop a deeper understanding of the pathogenesis of perverse symptoms. The focus is more on preoedipal, primarily nongenital anxieties which are specific to a particular stage of development and are linked to disturbances in the development of the self (Kohut 1973 a, b; Stolorow 1979; Morgenthaler 1974) or in object relationships (Winnicott 1958; Socarides 1960; Khan 1979).

The sexualization in the perversion has a stabilizing function: it relieves other nonsexual areas of the personality, for example by binding and giving expression to predominantly aggressive "instinctual" wishes, anxieties and impulses in the perversion. This ritualized relief enables the self to remain coherent and intact (Kohut 1973 a, b). The more fragile the narcissistic organisation, the more existentially vital the perversion becomes as an assurance of one's own existence: "I experience pleasure, hence I exist" (Eissler 1958, p. 239)

The perversion functions as a kind of "filling", as Morgenthaler (1974) described it, plugging a hole left in an ego disturbed in its narcissistic development, and so protects it from feelings of emptiness and futility. Glover (1956 also pointed out that the perversion's purpose is to paper over the cracks in the development of a sense of reality. Or, to use another image, the perversion is a kind of emergency bridge between archaic perceptions organized by primary thought processes and outward reality organized by secondary processes, so enabling the self to stabilize itself and achieve a sense of intactness. In the fenced-off area of the perversion magical primary thought processes can find expression and narcissistic tension can be discharged without endangering the person's foothold in reality. The "perverts have given the dictatorship of sexuality an island where it works off its urges so the rest of the dominion can be left undisturbed ... The perverse organization of sexuality secures the personality's emotional coherence by consuming all the influences that could block it" (Morgenthaler 1984, p. 36).

Besides these metapsychological conceptions of perversion, there is Stoller's concept (1975) which, being closer to clinical reality, emphasizes two important clinical aspects: we have Stoller to thank for pointing out that a characteristic rage and hatred form the specific and essential kernel of a perverse symptom or, as he wrote, the perversion is "an erotic form of hatred". Moreover, Stoller believes that a childhood drama lies hidden behind every perverse ritual, recalling the traumata suffered while trying to develop a male identity. A perverse phantasy or act is a scenario in which these traumata are reconstructed and re-enacted, but only in such a way that the early injuries and defeats can be momentarily denied; for an instant it is as if they had never been, and in their stead there is a euphoric sense of satisfaction and triumph. The weak point in this concept is not just that it is based in an almost behaviouristic way on the concrete, biographically traceable traumatic event and less on the "perennial emotional climate", but above all that Stoller confines the problems underlying perversion exclusively to male identity development, which usually forms only *one* aspect of the perverse symptom. Those involved tend very often to have more wide-ranging disturbances; the impairment of their male identity is then just one manifest aspect of a complex set of problems.

3.2.1.2 Clinical Aspects

Studies on sexual perversions all too easily give the impression that, despite the variety of possible meanings a perversion can have, one is dealing with a uniform phenomenon; they suggest there is a nosological entity perversion, which is by no means confirmed by clinical experience. On the contrary, one comes across an extraordinary variety in the way the perversion presents itself and its course of development. By this we do not mean the different patterns within which the perversion is acted out, which can be found in the usual classification (fetishism, sadomasochism, exhibitionism, etc.), but the widely different ways a perversion is anchored in the structure of personality and the relative importance of the role it plays. In clinical work it is important to delineate three aspects which are closely connected. They are important for diagnosis because they involve consequences for therapy. The three aspects are: the intensity and frequency of perverse acts, the role they play in the organisation of the psyche and how closely the perversion is related to the ego.

The Varying Intensity of Perverse Symptoms

Among sex offenders there is only a small minority which has developed a real sexual perversion in the sense of a stable, internal structure resulting in constant, sexually deviant orientation. A few are fetishists or pedophiles, less often voyeurs or exhibitionists; only rarely does a sadomasochistic perversion lead to a violent sexual offence. In a large majority of cases sexual offences are the expression of a momentary, sporadic or frequently recurring perverse impulse which only emerges in a particular situation or a critical phase of life and does not otherwise restrict the person's sexual orientation. In simplified terms, one can distinguish four different degrees of intensity:

1. A perverse impulse emerges only once or *sporadically* and is linked to a current conflict or a particularly critical situation in life. It is no longer felt after overcoming the crisis, not even in phantasies. Many sexual offenders belong to this group, above all adolescent offenders. The theoretically imprecise and misleading concept of the "sexual substitute act" belongs here.

2. The perverse symptoms, as perverse reactions, turn into a constantly recurring *habitual conflict-solving pattern* which can always be reactivated and breaks through in phantasies or impulses when inner stress and crisis situations arise, without in general affecting sexual orientation or sexual desires. Many recidivist exhibitionists, for example, belong to this group. It often proves possible to identify a link with psychological stress such as deeply hurt feelings or painful losses.

3. Real *perversion formation*, in the sense of stable deviant orientation, is far less frequent. Sexual desires and phantasies are not, or not intensely, experienced without perverse themes. The symptom has made itself more or less independent; in general, no connection to causative crises can be found.

4. *Developments and processes leading to an increase in severity* are particularly likely to occur in perversion formation. When an occasional or periodic enactment of the perverse ritual does not result in sufficient stabilization and relief, sexual needs and sexual phantasies occur more and more frequently and seep into more and more areas of life. Sexual needs are increasingly felt to be insistent and there is a subjective feeling that these impulses can no longer be resisted. This course of development was termed "sexual addictiveness" by Giese (1962). Giese identified certain characteristic "key symptoms": the "slide into sensuality", i.e. particular sensual stimuli acquire a signalling character; over time the frequency of perverse acts increases, while satisfaction decreases; there is a trend towards anonymity and promiscuity; and, finally, a specific inner state is reached which Giese termed "addictive experiencing".

These different levels of intensity can be explained by interpreting perverse symptoms psychodynamically. Depending on the intensity of the underlying anxieties, the severity of the conflict and the extent of the personality defect, defence behaviour proves more or less successful, with a lasting or short-term effect; stabilization via the perverse symptom succeeds, is unreliable, or hardly helps at all. The progressive proliferation of the perverse syndrome is a sign that the relief a perverse symptom provides is, or has become, insufficient. Internal tension increases; this always results in an increasingly frequent and more urgently sought and restless effort to find relief by continually repeating the perverse ritual, with less and less success.

The Significance of a Perversion in Personality Structure

Looking at the striking variations in the intensity of a perversion from another angle, we can ask to what extent a perverse symptom is circumscribed and can be isolated. With our procedure of first observing the perverse symptom and probing it for its psychological meaning and significance, we discovered when evaluating the project that this question was not always easy to answer. These difficulties cannot only be explained by the varying success we had in developing an empathic understanding for different patients. In fact, this phenomenon has its roots in distinct differences in patient structure. The degree to which a perverse symptom can be clearly separated from "nonperverse" elements in a personality structure can be summarized in three basic prototypes:

1. The classical case mostly discussed in perversion literature is that the *perverse symptom,* in analogy to other neurotic symptom formations, is *circumscribed* and follows a fixed ritual. Often in marked contrast to the remaining social personality, or at least separable from it, the symptom can be interpreted as a reparative enactment of a describable set of problems. Being "isolated from emotional experience", it appears as an "alien element in the personality" (Morgenthaler 1984); this "island" with its relief function is a "creative achievement of the ego" (see Cases 2, 6 and 15).

2. Among sexual delinquents the perverse symptom usually does not appear in a delineated, fixed, ritualized and periodically recurring form. This is more often the case with severely disturbed patients who, because of their fragmentary personality structure, are generally more defenceless against an upsurge of powerful instinctual drives. The dynamics in such cases are often extremely destructive; impulses are hardly under control and can break through in manifold, sometimes sexualized and often polymorphous perverse forms. They are what Schorsch and Becker (1977) described as "impulsive acts" or what Kernberg (1975) called "impulse neuroses" (see Case 18). Other less disturbed patients decompensate in acute, often age-specific crises in which they commit a (frequently aggressive) sex offence; this cannot, however, be regarded as a stable perverse symptom formation (see Case 5).

3. Finally, there are the very rare patients with a fully established, stable perversion which cannot be said to have a clearly delineated reparative function for definable gaps. In such cases the perversion is like a clasp holding the fragmentary structure together. It acts as a sheet anchor as the patients no longer have any compensatory, nonperverse coping strategies. The typical perverse mechanisms pervade more or less all areas of the personality. These can be termed *perverse character structures.* To use Morgenthaler's images, the "island" of perversion cannot be seen apart from the "rest of the land" in which it is meant to keep the peace. Only the island is still visible (see Case 7).

The Relation of the Perversion to the Ego

This aspect involves differences in the intrapsychic processes with which patients deal with their perverse symptoms on a more conscious level and the kind of relationship which exists between the perversion and the superego or ego ideal. There is a continuum here between the two poles *ego-syntonic* and *ego-dystonic. Ego-syntonic coping* means accepting the perverse symptom, integrating it into the concept of self and seeing it in a positive light. This is hardly ever found in sexual delinquents in its pure form and more often but not exclusively in convinced pedophiles who ideologically exaggerate their sexual orientation. At the other end of the scale, *ego-dystonic coping,* one finds patients who respond to their perverse symptom with a sense of shame, guilt feelings, anxieties of various kinds and intensity, who see it in a very negative light, cannot reconcile it with their self-image and suffer from it. One particular form of ego-dystonic coping takes the form of experiencing the extremely unwelcome symptom as something ego-alien which does not belong to them, like an illness that has befallen them. The perversion, which is actually a vital plug, is felt to be an isolated block which cannot be integrated into their self-image and for which ego ideal and superego are, so to speak, no longer responsible. The pure form of either ego-syntonic or ego-dystonic coping is scarcely ever seen in rea life; ego-syntonic and ego-dystonic aspects often exist side by side or the subject alternates between the two extremes.

3.2.2 Frequently Recurring Meanings of the Symptom

Our procedure here was as follows: we attempted to decode the meaning behind a perverse ritual by relating it to a central conflict pattern which we derived from the patient's development and life history. Set against this background, we were able to find different compensatory aspects in the symptom Initially, 32 cases were assessed using this method. Then, by inductively forming categories (see Sect. 3.1.2) we filtered out the seven typical thematic feature which had been listed most frequently in the previous step. The variety of possible symptom meanings is, of course, by no means completely covered by these seven aspects; in fact, this selection only reflects some aspects of a complex set of meanings and each symptom incorporates several of these aspects Listing them separately only makes sense if they are understood as comprising only part of the overall meaning.

Demonstrating Masculinity

The fact that the perverse act is momentarily accompanied by an intense feeling of potency, virility and power is one of the pivotal characteristics of mos perverse rituals. This indicates that an unstable male gender identity, an uncertainty about being a proper man, is an almost ubiquitous basic theme in thes patients. Most perverse symptoms are also an attempt to compensate an injur to male self-esteem, to restore a sense of manliness. In this respect one can agree with Stoller (1975). However, a perversion cannot generally be attributed just to a circumscribed masculinity problem. Far more frequently the reason lies in earlier and more fundamental disturbances which have impaired structural development in numerous different ways; a vulnerable male identity is then only one aspect among many others.

In the patients' biographies we repeatedly found circumstances which impeded identification with a father. Many patients grew up without a father (20% of the patients were born illegitimately) or their father played a minor role in family life compared with their dominating mother. A situation such as this prevents the male child from terminating his primary symbiotic identification with his mother (Greenson 1961) and so creating the foundation for the development of a stable feeling of masculinity. Later relationships may then be handicapped, for instance by fusion or separation anxieties which are warded off by a pronounced demonstration of phallic potency.

If the son experienced the father as negative, threatening or overpowering in his maleness - as was the case for quite a number of our patients - male identification may also be impeded. These fathers ridicule and reject their sons, either because - on the phallic level - they see them as rivals and are jealous or - on an oral level - because they are envious of the intimate, caring relationship between mother and child (see Klein 1932).

Symptoms which are a demonstration of masculinity are very often seen in exhibitionism and in violent attacks, in sadomasochistic assertion of power, but also in pedophile acts in which the age and power gap can be a central component in providing satisfaction: confrontation with the child's genitals gives pedophiles the feeling of being genitally potent and mitigates their doubts and anxieties about their own masculinity. In other pedophile acts which focus less on genitality and potency and more on a regressive escape into a child's world, this meaning may be completely absent.

Avoiding Genitality

This meaning behind the symptom, avoiding genitality, is the reverse of "demonstrating masculinity" and suggests a more pronounced masculinity problem which is coped with and expressed differently in the perverse ritual. While demonstrating masculinity can be interpreted as resorting to counterattack, a regressive avoidance of genital sexuality is found particularly in patients who mainly associate sexuality in their unconscious phantasies with being aggressive, dangerous and destructive, with having to prove themselves or with being castrated or annihilated. This is often what the symptom means in nonaggressive pedophile acts which entail regression to the infantile position. It is also found, however, in voyeurism, fetishism or even in some exhibitionists who associate exposing their genitals less with potency than with a gesture of abject impotence and subjugation and, for instance, always show their penis unerected, phantasizing women laughing at them for doing so (see Case 14). The following case illustrates what is meant by avoiding genitality.

Case 1

The 44 year-old patient came to us after a serious suicide attempt. He had been given a prison sentence, which had been suspended on the basis of a medical report, for sexually molesting his two adopted daughters.

The patient is seriously handicapped by a tracheostoma after a larynx operation. He is small, plain and looks older than he is. He tries to cover his noticeable embarrassment by being very friendly. His obligingness and willingness contain a defensive element and it is difficult to get beyond the level of mutual politeness.

He was an unwanted late child in a family which lacked warmth and affection. His father was a discontented, irascible man who once shouted at him: "I really shouldn't have brought you into the world." He was often beaten by both parents and was pushed around. As a child he was put in a home for 2 years, was then given to foster parents and later lived with his parents, brothers and sisters in a one-room apartment. After leaving secondary school he started, at his father's insistence, a painter's apprenticeship which he did not, however, complete. He then became a sailor and went to sea where he got along well. He fell in love with a girl in Venezuela. When her parents urged him to marry her, he "fled" back to his ship. Later he worked in a company and reached the position of department head.

He remembers at the age of 7 being lured into sexual games by his 14-year-old sister. She used to ask him to play with her genitals and he always had a strong sense of being cossetted and cared for in her warm bed. He was extremely shy with girls. His first sexual contacts took place after marriage at the age of 30; he suffered from erection and ejaculation dysfunctions which were very distressing for him and his wife. Being unable to have their own children, they adopted two daughters. His self-esteem was severely shaken because of his impotence and sterility. He withdrew from his wife and felt more and more unimportant and rejected by her. As the crisis came to a head, he committed incest with his adopted daughters to whom he had always had a very close emotional relationship. He displayed a very childlike sexual curiosity behaviour, playing a kind of doctor game in which genital sex and phallic potency played no role. When his wife found out about this from the children, the patient, who was completely desperate, made a serious suicide attempt with alcohol, pills and exhaust fumes. Afterwards he spent one and a half years in hospital and had to undergo surgery of the larynx several times as it had been damaged during reanimation intubation.

Psychodynamic Aspects: The patient's loveless and unsettled early childhood gave rise to an extremely unstable sense of self, pointing to a deeply depressive personality core. He experienced maleness, associated with his ill-tempered father, as dangerous and incompatible with his longing for understanding and shelter; at the same time he saw himself as physically impotent, worthless, unwanted and unloved. In the *symptom* a regressive avoidance of "adult" and, in his eyes, both dangerous and jeopardized phallic genital sexuality emerged. It was an attempt to re-enact the incestuous situation with his sister which he experienced as warm and protective and in which he could find consolation and approval.

Therapy: see p. 102.

Rage and Hatred

Like masculinity problems, aggressive feelings, including rage and hatred are, as Stoller (1975) emphasized, of central importance at a deeper level for the perverse symptom. This hatred is expressed on the one hand by depersonalizing the object and making it into a fetish in perverse phantasies or actions and on the other by feeling the triumph involved in reversing the roles and paying back earlier insults; this feeling, in Stoller's view, is what very specifically characterizes perverse pleasure.

The more vehemently the masculinity problem is acted out in the perverse symptom, the more obviously aggressive feelings come to the surface as rage and hatred, even though they may not be consciously experienced. On this deeper level, such rage is mostly directed against the mother as she is frequently experienced as someone who hindered any attempts to become autonomous and fully male. This meaning behind the symptom is not just confined to those perverse enactments in which (phallic) aggressive feelings are acted out as open violence, but is also found wherever such feelings are manifested symbolically as a threat (e.g. indecent exposure) or are concealed behind a seemingly peaceful passivity, as in some fetishists, voyeurs and a few pedophiles.

As well as the problem of maleness, this meaning points out another crucial aspect in these patients: the problem of (coping with) aggression. In the complex interplay of forces influencing the development of drive, object relations and self-awareness, early traumata give rise to the cracks or gaps in the personality structure mentioned above which, depending on the ego's functioning ability, are compensated on different levels. If in early developmental phases, for instance during the symbiotic phase between mother and child or during the critical separation phase, little empathy is available for the specific needs of the child, then the result can be that aggressive and/or destructive elements are poorly neutralized or integrated. These early traumatizations can turn out to be a serious handicap to negotiating the phallic phase successfully. Phallic-sexual and destructive impulses become contaminated by early anxieties (Greenacre 1952). The important adaptive function of developing a perverse symptom consists in the *protection of the object*. Current relationships are spared this non-integrated aggression, thanks to it being bound into the symptom (Bak 1953).

The problem of how to cope with aggressive impulses can manifest itself outside the perverse symptom in several ways: one extreme form is shown by those patients who show no sign of aggressiveness in either their social behaviour or their therapeutic interaction, and whose aggressive tendencies are exclusively compensated and integrated in the perverse symptom (see Case 6). The other extreme is shown by patients with a generally high aggression potential which can be expressed in other areas and in varying degrees, as well as in the perverse symptom. Between these two extremes there are all kinds of variations to be found.

Act of Defiance

This meaning behind the symptom differs from the others above in that it does not apply to the perverse symptom itself, but to specific circumstances. Characteristic is an extreme contrast between the life style and social personality, on the one hand, and perverse impulses which run free in the symptom on the other. These patients often live hemmed in by external constraints but also bound down by a rigid, narrowly defined inner scheme of order. Everything appears to be preplanned, there is little room for unpredictable, unplanned events or for spontaneity or liveliness. The patients comply, conform and orient themselves on outer expectations and rigid inner norms up to the point of seemingly losing their freedom, although they function socially. This state of affairs is frequent in exhibitionists.

Psychodynamically speaking, it is interesting that these patients tend to seek dependency in relationships, preferring, for example, dominating and exacting partners. An act of defiance then frequently functions as a protest against this confinement; it is a momentary experience of delightful liberation as an antithesis to the straitjacket of their rigid structures, a moment of escape from the iron grip they feel as a threat, particularly to their male identity. From time to time they burst their social bonds to preserve their autonomy by demonstrating their masculinity and aliveness. In addition to the intrapsychic rescue function, this outburst nevertheless contains another element: it helps to maintain the security and order created, which also provides shelter by canalizing the inner anger against the strict partner without jeopardizing the relationship. In this respect too the symptom has the function of protecting the object. The essentially irreconcilable maintenance of order and its repeated, momentary destruction is possible because the subject frequently experiences the perverse symptom as something split-off, ill and alien.

Case 2

The 38-year-old patient had been previously convicted several times for exhibitionist acts. He started treatment voluntarily.

The tall, carefully dressed patient makes a correct, well-controlled and friendly impression. He chooses his words carefully and seems to iron out inconsistencies in his thoughts before speaking. His exhibitionism is completely incomprehensible to him. His deep embarrassment makes him describe himself factually, as if he were an object.

He is the only son born after four daughters. The family was well-to-do, home life was marked by strict order, considerable pressure to make a success of things and religious fanaticism. His mother was in charge, his father drank frequently and then became aggressive. Nobody respected him. The patient has always regretted not having a brother in this women's household. He does not feel he was taken seriously by his sisters. After "confessing" with great difficulty to his mother of pains while urinating, he was operated for a phimosis when he was 9 years old. He experienced this operation as a mutilation. As an adult he is still unable to show himself naked because he feels inferior. To his parents' great disappointment he only completed secondary school, although he was intelligent, and subsequently took on a commercial apprenticeship. He broke off a promising career in the army when it became known that he exposed himself. Another promising career attempt failed for the same reason. It is typical of him that his wish to expose himself occurs just at the time when he seems to be heading for promotion. Periods of unemployment were extremely humiliating for him. He finally found employment as a commercial traveller and again soon gained much recognition.

In puberty he had extreme scruples about masturbating and anxieties owing to his "mutilated" penis. At 18 he had his first intimate contact with a woman 10 years older than himself. He married at 27; he usually leaves the sexual initiative to his wife. He remains passive and likes to be seduced. He feels controlled and hemmed in by his wife and often has the wish to break out. He does so by hanging around and drinking in the Hamburg dock area for whole nights, while slipping deeper into a mood of loneliness, inferiority, stress and fear of failure. In these moods he feels the need to expose himself. He finds it exhilarating to provoke curiosity, interest and attention. This is followed by powerful guilt feelings which in turn induce the wish to expose himself again.

Psychodynamic Aspects: The problem centres on an insecure male identity with easily revived anxieties of castration and failure; these stem from the weak father who could scarcely be an example or an identification figure for him amongst the women he felt were influential and scornful. The fear of failure recurs more strongly the more he can assert himself through competence at work. He is then overwhelmed by a fear of the heights he has attained. After making a good start he always fails again, as if he himself acts out his own castration and degradation, although he repeatedly manages to start again. It is particularly striking how his childhood situation reemerges in his marriage (dominant wife, her subordinate husband who periodically breaks free). On the one hand the *symptom* has the function of convincing this man, who fails because of success, that he is a powerful male, of allowing him to feel his phallus and of convincing him that his maleness is intact despite his "mutilation". On the other hand it enables him to attract the attention as a man that he missed in his upbringing in a "women's household". The symptom is also an escape from female dominance and derision, a triumph over women's rule, giving him briefly a sense of being very much alive and potent.

Therapy: see p. 78.

Omnipotence

Between the meaning "demonstrating masculinity" and the meaning "feeling omnipotent" behind the perverse symptom there is a marked qualitative difference. Feeling omnipotent we regard as a momentary regression reviving the infant's phantasies of omnipotence and grandeur. While demonstrating masculinity essentially is a means for coping with a masculinity problem ubiquitous in perversions, feeling omnipotent indicates a less frequent and more fundamental disturbance in the narcissistic organization of the personality. This aspect of compensating by demonstrating omnipotence was seen only in a quarter of our patients. The feeling of being impotent, insignificant and worthless, whether constantly present or only in crises, is banished in the perverse act by primitively overestimating phallic potency and experiencing the (sexualized) power linked with it. This meaning behind the perverse symptom, transforming experienced impotence into phantasised omnipotence, is mostly observed in violent sexual offences; it is pathognomonic, above all for sadomasochistic perversions (Schorsch and Becker 1977). These are generally severely disturbed patients who feel constantly threatened by relationships and who are struggling to establish or maintain their autonomy (see Cases 7, 9 and 18).

Filling Up an Inner Void

Lichtenstein (1970) has described the function that sexuality has in enabling a person to take a sensual pleasure in his own independent existence: "Sexuality constitutes the primary, most archaic and nonverbal mode through which the conviction of one's existence is affirmed as an incontrovertible truth" (p. 312). This aspect has special significance for our patients. In almost all the patients it became apparent that the perverse symptom was meant to act as consolation, to build up self-assurance and to fill up an inner void. When this is the essence of the symptom, it is likely that the patient suffers from a deep disturbance of the capacity to relate to others because of early internalization deficits and deprivation.

The symptom's reparative function lies in the fact that the patients can gratify their mostly pregenital needs and take them into their own hands by sexualizing them, thereby making themselves independent of an environment which they expect to disappoint them. The symptom thus becomes a substitute for human intimacy which is not available on the relationship level, and comes close to what Winnicott (1958) described as a "transitional object", which gives the infant the possibility of appeasing separation anxieties when its mother is away. Whilst a child, however, only has to rely temporarily on the illusionary transitional object during the critical phase of differentiating between self and object, patients with a deficient development of self need the perversion permanently to maintain their narcissistic equilibrium. At the same time the pleasure sought in the perversion creates an exhilarating feeling which can be of crucial importance in narcissistic crises for patients whose self-image is unstable. Both the narcissistic and the relationship aspects provide the patient with a *defence against depression*, enabling him to avoid feeling lonely, useless and empty. The perversion can also serve the purpose of warding off a depressive breakdown.

Wish Fulfilment Through Identification

The mechanisms of projective identification, described for the first time by Klein (1932), produce a pattern of relationships particularly typical of pedophile perversions. These are defence mechanisms such as splitting, projection and introjection used to overcome early separation anxieties. As the symbiosis dissolves, the child perceives different qualities, "object imagines" (Jacobson 1973) in the relationship to its mother. These early imagines and introjection of them protect it from feeling abandoned. The frustrating aspects of the mother-child relationship lead to the formation of "bad" mother imagines from which the child frees itself through projection; the gratifying, yielding aspects lead to "good" mother imagines which strengthen the self through introjection. The splitting or separation into good and evil imagines is necessary, owing to the still active destructive inner impulses to protect the good and keep it for oneself. Klein (1932) calls the phase of maintaining this split the "schizoid position".

These early mechanisms can return in pedophile perversions, where there is often a regressive re-enactment of the childhood situation. The act performed by the pedophile with the child is a fulfilment of his own wish. He identifies with the child and longs for tenderness, physical contact, to be pampered and protected, to feel his genitals lovingly accepted, etc. In the pedophile act there is fusion with the childhood alter ego into which the patient can project feelings or aspects of his own which are otherwise unbearable – such as feeling void, superfluous, weak, starved of affection. In the complex interlocking of simultaneous identification – with one's own needs projected into the children on the one hand, and with the quasi ideal, caring parent figures, on the other – highly idealized sexualized relationships can develop which are frequently legitimated by ideological overevaluation. This relationship pattern is found mostly in homosexual pedophiles. Besides wish fulfilment through identification, the pedophile situation helps to increase self-esteem and gratifies narcissistic needs owing to the adult's superiority over the child.

Violent pedophile acts represent compact processes in which qualitatively quite different aspects of the early mother-child relationship are revived and often exist side by side without interacting: aggressive impulses are often bedded in tender emotions and the transition from one to the other is abrupt. The disconnected existence side by side of contradictory aspects in the relationship is the result of projective identification: projection and identification with the good mother introjects create a lovingly tender, erotic relationship towards the child; the caring, tender, protective elements of the early mother-child relationship, as it were the good mother introjects, are at work here. The violent acts are activities of the evil, or bad mother introjects. An oscillating, faltering and unstable identification develops, in which the pedophile for a moment identifies with the "evil" mother and an instant later with the alarmed child, only to feel the evil mother again seconds later. The following case illustrates this situation.

Case 3

The 28-year-old patient with a trial pending came for therapy because of sexual acts with boys.

The patient is tall and makes a clumsy and awkward impression. He presents himself in a submissive and not very amiable manner and signals a helplessness which he tries very awkwardly to conceal.

He still lives at home. His parents were extremely strict throughout his childhood and adolescence and still keep a close eye on him today. There is a complete lack of affection at home and the family obeys rigid norms. His mother is not really interested in him, his father does not accept him and keeps telling him he is a good-for-nothing. He lives as a kind of outsider in the family and shuts himself off from the others. He remembers being deeply affected by the birth of his only brother when he was 12. He remembers how much attention his brother and the children of a cousin received, especially when they were ill. He is still very jealous of his brother nowadays, full of resentment, envy and hatred. He cannot control these impulses very well, and tends to lose his temper very easily. As a child he limped for a while as a result of having polio myelitis. At school he had difficulty fitting in. He was considered peculiar, was teased and beaten and had no friends or playmates. After leaving elementary school, he took a job with the German Railway Company. He often gets into trouble at work, quarrels with colleagues, is considered hot-headed and is often drunk. The reason behind his outbursts is that he is again the victim of teasing which has made him so distrustful that he feels all his colleagues' reactions are directed against him. Owing to his conspicuous behaviour he is constantly in danger of being fired. This, however, he denies and talks about being promoted. At home he is compliant and completely under his parents' control. The only emotional relationship he has is with his German shepherd bitch. On holiday or in his leisure time he goes skin diving ("submerging") and shooting.

He has not yet had any erotic relationships. At about 12 (birth of his brother) he began masturbating as a way of consoling himself. He has strong inferiority phantasies about his genitals. When his brother was 4 years old, the patient developed a sadomasochistic pedophile perversion with clearly anal tendencies which gradually took shape in his phantasies over the years. He mostly pictures himself in a childhood setting playing doctor with small boys. He imagines the boys are ill. He measures their temperature rectally and gives them enemas. He also has phantasies, however, of hitting the boys on their bottoms and aggressively penetrating their anus. He mostly phantasizes in the active, less often in the passive role.

Psychodynamic Aspects: This is a severe, primarily narcissistic personality pathology. The patient's generally negative image of self cannot be compensated by secret, defiant phantasies of being powerful; there is a considerable potential for narcissistic anger and envy which are easily activated due to the lack of structure, and can quickly shatter his weak impulse control. Behind the anal character traits there are oral dependency wishes which he tries to gratify partly by means of alcohol, partly through masochistic submission. Given his paranoid tendencies, he tends to retreat into himself and his (sexual) phantasies – a withdrawal which suggests lack of a firm foothold in reality.

The *perverse symptom* finds its scenario in the child/doctor games. The problem here is not one of masculinity, but essentially the regressive re-enactment of the childhood situation. In the pedophile perversion his envy becomes a major motif as a sign of an early, ungratified craving for love and attention. The mechanism of projective identification, with its constant oscillation between the good and the bad, is particularly obvious here: on the one hand he identifies with the ill, helpless children he looks after and heals, acting as the good mother; and, on the other, he also acts out the bad elements of the mother-child relationship when in his phantasies he sadistically torments, dominates and destroys the children – and, by identification, himself in the children – with a concomitant feeling of power and omnipotence enabling him to dispose of them at will. The symptom thus becomes a vehicle for his hatred of both his mother and his brother.

The symptom is not a perverse reaction, but the expression of a fixed and firmly established pedophile sadomasochistic perversion. There is no identifiable, sharp dividing line between the magical world of the perversion and his social personality. Anal-sadistic character traits pervade most of his personality. The perversion seems to be the area in which he can best sense that he is truly alive in contrast to his inner void.

Therapy: see p. 122.

3.3 The Problems Underlying a Perverse Symptom

We started out with the assumption that a psychodynamic understanding of perverse symptoms is of fundamental importance in diagnosis and therapeutic procedure. Having identified various aspects of the meaning and purpose of the symptoms we can now concretize this hypothesis.

Our seven interpretative symptom features indicate that the problems underlying symptoms are anchored especially in four areas or aspects of personality. In other words, there are essentially four aspects of personality disturbance which are manifested in the perverse symptom, where they are cushioned, balanced and compensated: 1) a *masculinity problem* or *disturbances in male identity,* 2) an *aggression problem,* 3) a *disturbance in narcissistic development* and 4) *relationship problems.* In more theoretical terms one can say that the scenario of a perverse symptom can be viewed from three perspectives: the *drive aspect* (male identity and aggression), the *aspect of object relations* (relationship/intimacy problems) and the *narcissistic aspect* (self-experience) (Table 4).
This classification, derived from interpretations of the perverse symptom should only be used as an aid to diagnosis and not be misused as an inflexible system. We find it useful as it is flexible enough to leave room for the extraordinary variety and heterogeneity to be seen in each case. Just as in a specific perverse symptom one meaning may be pronounced, another less evident or even

Table 4. Interrelation between symptom meaning and basic problem

Meaning of perverse symptom	*Basic problem*
Demonstrating masculinity Avoiding genitality	→ Male identity
Rage and hatred Act of defiance Omnipotence	→ Aggression
Filling up an inner void	→ Narcissistic aspect (self-experience)
Wish-fulfilment through identification	→ Capacity to relate to others

missing completely, a disorder or problem may well emphasize one aspect more than another. Moreover, it is important to remember that a disorder may be very differently weighted in each area affected. For the sake of a structure and to enable our diagnostic assessments to be evaluated statistically, we subdivided the four disturbance areas into a three-step scale: slight/moderate/severe. We shall attempt to relativize the lack of differentiation in this rather crude quantifying classification with case examples which illustrate the psychogenetic and psychodynamic dimensions.

3.3.1 Male Identity

The concept male identity covers three complementary aspects to which Stoller (1968) gave three different names: first, "core gender identity" which designates the elementary consciousness of (male) gender as an indispensable component of the concept of self. The second element is "gender identity" which essentially describes the conviction of embodying the (male) sex role with all its cultural implications, such as stereotype sex-role notions of social potency. The third aspect is gender identity in the sense of sex, having confidence in genital adequacy and potency. Whereas core gender identity posed no problems for our patients, their notions of social potency and, above all, sexual adequacy were pervaded by anxieties and feelings of inferiority.

On a more *phenomenological level* the masculinity problems and anxieties of these patients are as a rule concentrated in a *fear of adult women* or female sexuality which is more or less conscious in some and warded off in others. This forms something akin to a common denominator underlying the perverse symptoms.

Seen from a *psychodynamic angle* these anxieties can have various origins. At first sight it looks as though *castration anxiety* triggered by oedipal conflicts is generally extremely strong in men with perverse symptoms. There are indeed patients whose perverse symptoms can essentially be attributed to an oedipal castration anxiety of this kind (see Case 15). They are patients with a circumscribed masculinity problem; the failure to overcome oedipal conflicts is shown by the way the maturation processes in this phase remain rudimentary or incomplete: male identity and masculine sexual behaviour continue to be a problem and relations with women are still dominated by infantile fears and conflicts.

However, hidden behind the seemingly more superficial fear of castration anxiety in the majority of these patients there are deep anxieties which date from earlier stages of development. During the phallic narcissistic phase, faced with the oedipal triangle, *early anxieties* can be reactivated which reinforce the castration anxiety of this phase. We have described four such early anxieties (Becker and Schorsch 1980) which play an important role in this masculinity problem:

1. *Annihilation anxiety and fear of the ego's own dissolution* which originate in the active, projective identification with the mother in the early symbiotic phase. Deeply felt anger and hatred trigger archaic fears of dying, being destroyed or annihilated.

2. *Separation and fusion anxieties* are the consequence of an incomplete anal development; autonomy is inadequate and aggressive impulses have not been successfully neutralized. This makes separation from the mother almost impossible. The temptation to regress and merge with the maternal object simultaneously mobilizes immense fears, as this would involve being annihilated and losing oneself altogether.

3. *Fear of losing control* as a symptom of insecure (anal) impulse control on the one hand, and as an expression of alarm because of undefused aggressive impulses on the other.

4. *Body image anxieties* affecting the body, its wholeness and intactness. In contrast to castration anxieties, these are rooted in the development of the body image in the anal phase.

These early anxieties, which can share the common denominator "fear of woman" and form the basis of a fragile male identity, may vary from patient to patient and differ greatly in their significance. This explains the great structural heterogeneity hidden behind such labels as "masculinity problem, fragile male identity".

Using a scale, we assessed how vulnerable the patients' sense of maleness was. At the lowest level of disturbance identity we put those patients who had developed a basically sound *male identity*, but whose confidence in full genital adequacy and (social) potency proved easily *disturbed*. In crises and frustrating situations anxieties were mobilized which then had to be compensated by various defence processes, such as acting out the perverse symptom. In pathological terms, these patients have problems which mainly stem from an oedipal castration anxiety and doubts about their masculinity (see Cases 2 and 15). About one fifth of our patients fit into this category.

Patients whose confidence in their maleness was deeply shaken, whose *male identity* was noticeably *unstable and fragile*, not necessarily associated with any particular psychological crisis, were rated as being moderately disturbed. We assigned about half of our patients to this category. In developmental terms, pre-oedipal anxieties of various kinds play a role here.

Case 4

We were asked for an expert opinion on this 39-year-old Arab senior engineer as he had forced his way into women's apartments, exposed himself, and then attacked the women. He had been prosecuted for 11 such incidents.

This personable, cultivated patient seems to be in a sombre, depressive state of mind. He is deeply ashamed and full of guilt feelings, tight-lipped, but meticulously polite. It is difficult to talk to him. His distrustful, if not paranoid expression evokes uneasiness but also pity.

He comes from a well-to-do and influential family which holds key positions in society. Even nowadays he is still full of hatred towards his aloof, irritable and strict "superfather" from whom he suffered during his childhood and adolescence. He was the only one among his many brothers and sisters who dared to stand up to him, which only led to more punishment. His memories of childhood focus on his circumcision at the age of 6, an event he experienced as violent castration. Being more sensitive and gentler than his brothers, he feels like a eunuch. He is deeply attached to his mother but sees her as someone unable to exert any influence on family life. He was the only one in the large family to leave home at 18 for West Germany. For him this represented a final break with his home and past. Being culturally alien, he had great difficulty accustoming himself to the new environment. He went to university, was ambitious, worked in various jobs in good positions and eventually became self-employed. He invests an enormous amount of effort in his career to prove that he really is capable of something.

He was given a strict Mohammedan education which taught him to be ashamed of and ignore his body. His first sexual arousal during puberty provoked considerable anxiety; even nowadays he is still very shy of his body in general. He avoided making any contact with women for a long time and entertained the notion that he was impotent – initially a self-fulfilling prophecy. Later on he still did not lose his latent anxiety about his potency. He first exposed himself after surprising his first fiancée with another man: in a fit of rage at this woman he showed her his penis to humiliate and besmirch her.

At the age of 25 he met his present wife. She comes from a large, wealthy and closely knit family. He sought, as it were, refuge in a family union which resembled his own family. Although he did not admit it, his self-confident wife's tendency to see marriage more as a partnership collided with his Arab values, despite his respect for her. He tried to make up for this "dethronement" by making possessive demands on her, keeping a jealous watch over her. He was afraid he could not satisfy her sexually.

During the last few years the conflicts have escalated: their only child (a son) has behavioural disorders and the patient recognizes himself in him. His work is getting on top of him. His wife increasingly resists his attempts to supervise her and his patronizing manner. All of this has thrown him off balance: he complains of headaches, stomach pains, unrest, insomnia and trouble with his heart; from time to time he drinks alcohol, loses control of himself, is bad-tempered and is tempted to commit suicide. His sense of shame has prevented him ever really talking to anyone about his deviant sexuality. He hints at the existence of voyeuristic and exhibitionist problems over recent years, but then recants, unable to talk about the subject. He denies that his offences have any sexual motives, although they are quite unmistakeable. Instead he has built up an apparently paranoid relief system. He reports anonymous, threatening phone calls hinting that his wife is deceiving him. He broke into the apartments where he committed the offences because he had received anonymous hints that his wife was there with another man.

Psychodynamic Aspects: This patient's problem has roots dating from infancy in the paternal masculinity ideal which he experienced as extremely threatening. This culturally specific concept of unlimited male power and dominance over women, combined with the events he experienced in childhood as destructive and castrating, has led to the development of an insecure male identity. This patient is nonetheless a good example of someone with early and deep anxieties concealed beneath or even immersed in castration anxieties on an oedipal level. His compulsively rigid structure and lack of impulse control in moments of crisis point to problems on the anal level; body image anxieties help to undermine his fragile male identity. His paranoid structure, the multiple psychosomatic symptoms, his depressive moods and suicidal tendencies, his fears of dying and being annihilated all point to early disturbances which have contributed to his anxieties about his maleness.

For this patient, masculinity is closely associated with violence. After emigrating and escaping from his father, he was at first able to sustain his self-esteem through success at work; but then it collapsed when he was deceived by his fiancée. This confirmed his sense of being inadequate and sexually inferior and triggered the symptoms discussed here which he resorted to in crises: in the *symptom* he identifies with his father's aggressive masculinity and then feels powerful, potent and independent. He triumphs over his feeling of being castrated and takes revenge on the women who he feels have debased and deceived him. The symptom also contains elements of an escape from rigid conventions and the oppressive bond with his wife, without this bond being jeopardized.

Therapy see page 104.

Patients with *hardly any* (or as yet no) *perceptible male identity* are rated as being severely disturbed; they seem rather (pre-)pubertal or childish. They formed a good quarter of our patients.

Case 5

We saw this 26-year-old patient for the first time after he had been charged with committing rape. During his 2 1/2 years of imprisonment his wife and mother had done their very best to get him therapy. Persuasive phone calls and numerous court applications preceded therapy. When his wife's interest gradually subsided, his mother took the initiative and pretended she was his wife when making telephone enquiries. The patient developed a cardiac neurosis, threatened to commit suicide and was repeatedly admitted to psychiatric wards.

The patient is small, slightly thickset, red-cheeked, smartly dressed and makes a childlike, pliant and very helpless impression. He looks like someone who wants to be taken by the hand, or even better, in someone's arms. He is plaintive, feels he is the victim of hostile circumstances and his appeals for help contain an element of blackmail.

He has a lower middle-class background. His parents' marriage is bad. He does not feel any affection for his father. He has always had a very close relationship to his mother who pampers and looks after him as much as she can and would like to follow his every footstep. They understand each other "without words". Earlier on he was jealous of his brother (10 years younger), but not later when he realized that the close bond with his mother was not affected by his brother. As a child he was shy, tongue-tied, easily embarrassed, anxious and frequently had headaches. After leaving elementary school he completed an apprenticeship as a joiner. He was in steady employment until he was arrested. In his occasional relationships with girls, who generally took the initiative, he was uncertain about his potency. Until marriage at the age of 23, he lived with his mother whose attention he increasingly felt to be restrictive and suffocating, without admitting as much. This relationship is double-edged: he feels incapable of getting on without her, enjoys being spoilt by her materially; on the other hand, he hates her as he feels handicapped by her, is unable to do anything on his own and always feels her watchful eye on him. This state of affairs did not change when he married, which was an attempt to escape from his mother's influence. His wife is not very independent either and is rather childish. Both remain in very close contact with their parents who interfere with everything.

Since puberty he has masturbated several times a day, even after marrying. Occasionally he has rape phantasies in which he breaks down the girls' defences so that they are docile and submit to his wishes. A few days before marrying he raped a young girl. He committed his second rape immediately after the birth of his son. He says that in both cases the girls agreed to what he was doing.

Psychodynamic Aspects: The patient has a very immature personality; owing to the protracted bond with his indulgent and interfering mother he did not develop a male identity and remained in a symbiotic, childlike dependency on her. He views his environment from the point of view of his own needs, is unable to empathize and delegates responsibility for his actions onto other people who he uses for his own interests. Compulsive masturbation offers an opportunity to feel momentarily that he has a separate and individual identity, to compensate for feeling helpless and dependent on his possessive mother. Violent outbursts occur in situations in which he makes commitments and assumes responsiblity (marriage, birth of child) and his anger with women comes to light. This also makes it quite clear that the real problem does not lie primarily in oedipal influences (the close, eroticized mother-child relationship). Rather, the core of the problem seems to lie in fears of separation and fusion, triggering his rage against his mother who has obstructed his autonomy. In the *symptom* he changes roles: from the weak, docile and unmanly victim he feels himself to be, he is transformed into a potent, powerful man who overwhelms women and renders them defenceless.

Therapy see p. 90.

3.3.2 Aggression

Just as with the disturbances in the development of a male identity, it is important to distinguish the *psychogenetic influences* and the origins of the aggressive behaviour: whether the impulses are more oral-sadistic or anal-sadistic in nature, whether they are the expression of a "narcissistic rage" (Kohut 1973a) or rather of phallic aggressive origin. Diagnostically it is important to know from which anxieties mentioned in the last section the aggressiveness stems and, furthermore, whether and how the aggressive impulses are integrated in the self-image.

We can leave aside the current controversy in psychoanalysis as to whether aggression is an inborn, "instinctual" or reactive process, or both. It is indisputable that "aggression is activated by any impedance of satisfaction of libidinous and narcissistic (self-)needs" (Mentzos 1982). Diagnostically aggression can, on the one hand, be assigned to the *anxieties* discussed above, inherent in the phases of psychosexual development and, on the other, as a force to be integrated in the course of *autonomy development.*

The deeper and earlier *anxieties* are anchored, the greater is the aggression potential. The easier it is to mobilize fears, for example, of being annihilated and destroyed, the greater becomes the control a person needs to hold his or her destructive anger in check. In clinical work with our patients we noticed that even minor insults, disappointments or frustrations sufficed to spark off highly destructive or autodestructive behaviour, sometimes within and sometimes outside the symptom.

This more reactive element in the service of defence against infantile anxieties is supplemented by another aspect furthering the *development of autonomy*: one prerequisite for developing a stable sense of self, which later enables the person to relate to others without too much anxiety, is successful separation from the mother-child symbiosis, which includes giving up the primary identification with the mother. Aggression is needed to make this separating step, in which it is neutralized and channelled into independence, the ability to take the initiative and choose for oneself, to develop curiosity and take pleasure in one's own competence. If this step is impeded, aggression retains its oral-destructive components which are later manifested in uncontrolled outbursts or depressive reactions - phenomena which we often observed in our patients. In the therapeutic setting, this means the patients have to start coping with their aggressive feelings while separating themselves step by step from the therapist.

When assessing how aggressive our patients were, another central criterion, besides the biography and the way the patients presented themselves, was whether and to what extent aggressive behaviour was *noticeable in the therapeutic interaction*. At first we found, to our surprise, that at least one quarter of our patients *did not show any signs of aggression*. It was not even noticeable in the countertransference in the form of uneasiness, impatience, irritability, discomfort, etc. Such patients scarcely show any sign whatsoever of normal and healthy aggressive elements in their social behaviour and seem to have an aggression defect. In therapy they mostly make a naive, trusting impression; they are likeable but seem to lack profile and are not easy to come to grips with; since they do not offer any resistance, it is difficult to have a constructive discussion. However, this does not preclude their aggressive potential manifesting itself elsewhere than in social relationships, e.g. in (sexual) phantasies and/or (sexual) symptoms. Another 10% of our patients were assessed to have a very low level of aggressiveness. This means that more than one third of the patients were distinctly "aggression inhibited" in social contexts, at least as far as expressing aggressive impulses in socially acceptable ways was concerned.

Case 6

This 24-year-old patient was sent for treatment after being tried for indecent exposure to women. He had been convicted five times since the age of 16.

He acts like a boy who has been up to mischief, ruefully admits it and is likely to get off lightly because he is such an honest, well-behaved and good fellow. He has a disarming way of winning over others in his favour.

His mother died when he was 3 years old. For a few years he lived with his grandmother until his father married again and took him back. He did not feel close to him and his stepmother. His father was strict and expected a lot of him. His two younger half-sisters were always presented to him as an example of how he should be. He felt lonely and isolated in the family, but always fitted in so that friction and conflicts never arose. As his schoolwork deteriorated he was sent to boarding school at 10. He was not home-sick and fitted in well. He was forced to leave boarding school at 16 after he had exposed himself for the first time. He has been interested in music from an early age and went to train as a violin maker.

Since he otherwise always adapted to others, for him sexuality was something that he secretly reserved for himself; he was deeply fascinated by it. He often masturbated during puberty and was preoccupied by sexual phantasies and daydreams. He was shy of girls, failed to make contact and thought his penis was too small. He exposed it for the first time at the age of 15. In doing so, his wish was to seduce girls, but not to frighten them. He says that girls accepted his showing his penis as an offer of contact and slept with him. These memories still delight him today. Even when women ask him why he does things like that and involve him in a discussion he is not at all embarrassed, but considers this a success. He enjoys exciting attention.

His sexual experiences before marriage were restricted to visiting brothels which he found sobering and disappointing. At 21 he met his future wife in the church choir. She is domineering, his superior and takes little sexual interest in him. He cannot get his sexual wishes across to her and feels rejected by her. Like his parents earlier, she expects a lot of him. She is dissatisfied with his level of education and urges him to earn more. He has the feeling he is not getting anything in return from her. He has continued to expose himself frequently and regularly during the marriage and conceals this from his wife.

Psychodynamic Aspects: After having lost his mother early on, the patient was forced to adapt to changing parent figures and situations. His lack of sensibility, combined with a childish, naive confidingness typical of him, are evidence of poorly developed autonomy and of an extremely unstable self-image. He constantly has to adapt and does so indiscriminately, while denying his own and others' aggressive impulses in order to be noticed at all and given some attention. The *symptom*, in which he identifies with his penis, has the function of re-establishing his narcissistic equilibrium. In his phantasy it makes him confident of being vivacious, interesting and attractively virile and is at the same time embedded in his naive courting behaviour.

Therapy see p. 89.

In a good quarter of our patients *aggression* rated as *unremarkable*. This applies to patients who can get their own way and assert themselves; they respond in an appropriately resolute manner to their environment. In terms of masculinity they have a fairly well developed, though susceptible male gender identity.

When rating a further third as *markedly aggressive* we do not primarily mean they behave more aggressively, but above all that the aggressiveness has a different quality; it frequently has a destructive tendency and is also often difficult to control because it has not been neutralized or adequately integrated into their self-image. Such aggressive impulses can be either open or concealed, and directed outwards or inwards at themselves. Autodestructive aggression then makes itself felt in the therapeutic interaction, not as fear *of* the patient, but as fear *for* the patient. This means that besides the patients with severe aggression inhibition, there is an equally large group with a high potential for behaving aggressively, whose impulse control is low and who often experience the eruption of aggressive impulses as ego-alien and frightening (see Case 18).

3.3.3 Narcissism

Running parallel to the development of object libido, and its phase-specific relationship patterns between mother (father) and child, there are other processes which promote *narcissistic development*. These are closely linked with drive and ego development. The starting point is the state of primary narcissism in the first few weeks of life. The more the original narcissistic balance starts to waiver and the symbiosis weakens, the more the child develops archaic phantasie: aimed at preserving the feeling of being complete and at restoring the origina invulnerability. Kohut (1973 a, b) describes in particular two kinds of archaic im ages which he calls narcissistic configurations: first, illusions of grandeur witl which the child protects itself from fears of being detached from its mother These notions temporarily give the child a sense of being immensely powerfu and independent. The second narcissistic configuration consists of the ideal ized parent image which enables the child to share in their parents' power an(importance by identifying with them. These basic configurations are later trans formed and integrated into structures closer to reality – such as superego, ego ideal, ego-syntonic ambitions and purposes – and form the foundation of : positive image of self and body. Any disturbances in this narcissistic develop ment always reveal themselves in the manner the person experiences himself.

When assessing how someone experiences himself, his self-image, the mai criteria are the reliability and stability of his self-perception, and regulation o his self-esteem, trust in his own values and an accepting attitude towards hi own body. As might be expected, doubts about their own worth and a sense o insecurity are common in these patients, but they vary greatly in form and in tensity.

For just under half of the patients the *negative aspects of self-image* or fluctu ations in their self-perception have *little influence* or can for the most part b *compensated* by positive aspects (see Cases 14, 15).

In contrast, one fourth of the patients have a thoroughly *negative self-imag* their basic attitude towards life is a compound of worthlessness, futility, empt ness, depression and self-contempt (see Cases 10 and 16). One important aspe(of a negative self-image, particularly in these patients, is a rejecting and depre ciating attitude towards their own body.

In one fifth of the patients the self-image is discordant, expressed in extrem fluctuations in the way they perceive themselves; feelings of being worthles: helpless, nonexistent and despicable alternate with irrational notions of gra deur and might. These elements can exist independently side by side (se Case 4). It is rare for illusions of grandeur and omnipotence phantasies to tak the upper hand. These patients' general sense of impotence and futility is s pronounced that they have to escape into an almost incomprehensible gra diosity.

Case 7

This 30-year-old student of chemistry sought counselling on his own initiative. He has alrea(attempted and discontinued different kinds of therapy which he speaks of in highly derogat ry tones. However, he immediately tries to win over the therapist by handing out praise in a vance: he has at last found the right person who will definitely help him. It soon becomes e dent that not exhibitionism, but the risk of being punished is his main problem. He proud reports never having been caught, but is afraid that this will not last much longer as his ne(to expose himself is getting more and more out of control.

The patient is small, quick-witted and eloquent. He makes a very self-assured impressi and lets one know straight away that he is someone special, so that only an outstanding the apist will be able to help him. He wants to impress his audience with his descriptions of himself; he behaves in an exhibitionist manner. Signs of weakness, helplessness and self-rejection only emerge once in a while and are then rapidly covered up.

He tells an unusual and amazing story: he is the son of a wealthy South American landowner of German origin and a Swedish actress. His parents used to quarrel all the time. His father was short-tempered and jealous and often beat up his mother. His mother paid more attention to his sister (2 years younger). His mother then left her husband, taking her daughter with her. He stayed with his father and felt "abandoned by two women who had disappointed me". He was often thrashed by his father, and at 14 experienced his father's death as a liberation. He then joined his mother in Sweden, but did not feel at home there either. In secondary school he tried to make a big impression on others, but was nonetheless an outsider. At 24 he moved to the FRG and started studying. He began to find it difficult to concentrate on work, and he became increasingly restless as his sexual problem grew. He earned his living by teaching languages.

The description of his sexual development plays a central role in his account of himself. He experiences all relationships as being sexually tinged. He repeatedly sketches memories of impressing others with his genitals, for example when his grandmother saw his erect penis and fled screaming from the room. He reiterates with childish pride that he has a particularly beautiful and impressive penis. Protracted exhibitionist and voyeuristic activities preoccupied him during childhood and puberty. In his descriptions phantasy and reality seem to intermingle. As an adolescent he boasted about womanizing, inventing all the stories. He has an image of himself as "Casanova" and believes others admire him for this. Since the age of 20 he has had numerous, usually fleeting, often simultaneous heterosexual relationships. It is important to him that these women admire him. Below the surface he is full of anxieties and inferiority feelings. He only chooses women who are intellectually and socially inferior and speaks about them disparagingly. At the start of therapy he had been living for the first time with a girlfriend for quite a while. This relationship reflects the problem: she is inferior to and dependent on him; he sees her as small and weak and she absolutely adores him - or so he says. He only needs her for her admiration but at the same time despises her for her weakness. Sex with her is becoming less and less exciting. He "picks up" other women, masturbates several times a day and is almost exclusively preoccupied with his exhibitionist ritual.

Psychodynamic Aspects: This patient's main problem is to be found in a severe narcissistic *character pathology,* i.e. a disturbance in his self-image characterized by a complete sexualization of his real and phantasy behaviour and feelings. By fixating on an infantile grandiosity he can defend himself against feeling helpless and inferior and can ward off any doubts about his masculinity. This patient's perversion cannot be seen as a separately definable symptom as the sexualization affects all areas of life. We prefer to term this a "perverse character structure". The whole pathology is concentrated in exposing the phallus, which becomes a substitute for the personality as a whole, a means of communication, the counterpart to his inner emptiness, expression of his potency and his contempt and hatred for the disappointing women.

Therapy see p.97.

3.3.4 Interpersonal Relations

Lichtenstein (1970) reports that "clinical observations do not confirm a clear correlation between emotional maturity (i.e. the capacity to establish stable object relations) and the ability to obtain full satisfaction through genital orgasm (genital primacy)" (p.317). Analysis of our patient group confirms this. Some patients have stable partner relationships despite their sexual difficulties (Case 14) and others, having no partner, can be potent and are capable of orgasm in short-lived contacts despite perversion (Case 13). The problem here i that genital sexuality is not integrated into adult love relationships. The path t achieving this is paved with "innumerable pitfalls" (Blanck and Blanck 1974) Maturation deficits are revealed especially in the quality of relationships – an this is important for therapy as the problem recurs in the therapist-patient rela tionship.

Those patients who are able to relate to a partner need their perverse symp tom to compensate for their doubts about their potency, stemming from castra tion anxieties. These patients usually have a stable inner structure. Most of ou patients lacked this ability to engage in emotionally mature relationships. Th prerequisite for the ability to love is an undisturbed symbiosis, followed by suc cessful separation and individuation (see Bergmann 1971; Bak 1971; Kernber 1975). The mourning processes to be coped with in separation, which also in volves giving up real childhood objects, lead to a sense of independence whic for the first time enables the person to feel concern and empathy as well a guilt feelings (Kernberg 1976). It became apparent in many of our patients tha the separation phase had been problematic; either they were still dependent o infantile love objects or – where the symbiosis had been dissolved too early they had been forced to become autonomous, leading later to a general mis trust which permitted at best a narcissistic relationship pattern (see Cases 1 and 13). Where detachment from the symbiosis had proved impossible, the re sult was object relationships of a pregenital nature which are also always a sig of ego weakness; they are characterized by "the persistence of infantile hope and expectations going far beyond what is really possible" (Balint 1952 p. 356). Balint assigned these immature relationships three characteristics: "de spondent dependence, denial of this dependence by 'omnipotence' and takin the object for granted, treating it as a mere object, as a thing ... That is wh this 'omnipotent' or 'greedy' love is unstable, doomed to meet with frustratio and to lead on to hate" (p. 357).

The relationship patterns of our patients reflect the pathological fixation rooted in the anxieties described: the partners are clung to, dominated, ideal ized, degraded, abandoned, functionalized, etc. We shall come across these pa terns again in the therapist-patient relationship.

When using our rough and ready scale, we have disregarded this dimensio of qualitative relationship structures and instead assessed the degree of *abili to relate* as an overall characteristic, i.e. the ability to enter into and maintai stable emotional relationships. According to our assessment the ability to ente into relationships was significantly impaired in all but about one fifth of ou patients (see Cases 2 and 15), and was seriously impaired in about half of th patients; the way in which they structure relationships is so abnormal and im mature that relationships fail to stabilize. This problem was even more pro nounced in about one third of the patients. Attempts to form relationship failed from the very beginning; in extreme cases we observed an apparently au tistic complete lack of attachments (see Cases 9 and 18).

3.4 The Intensity of the Disturbance and Personality Pathology

When describing the various aspects of a symptom, its meaning and significance in Chap. 3 we touched on the question of the severity of the pathology. In presenting the four typical problem areas: male identity, the problem of aggression, narcissistic aspects of the self-image and difficulties in relating to others, we assessed the levels of intensity for each of them, using a slight/medium/severe scale. None of these partial aspects can however serve alone as indicator of how severe a personality pathology is; this can, in fact, only be established by taking all the aspects into account. Particularly for statistical reasons we have made a synoptic, overall assessment of personality pathology according to the intensity and severity of the disturbance.

Patients who fell into the *group of least disturbed,* "healthiest" patients were those whose male identity was considered to be fairly well established even though it remained vulnerable, who did not have a serious aggression problem, whose narcissistic self-image was fairly consistent and whose ability to relate was not severely impaired. These are patients where the perverse symptom is more or less circumscribed and serves to back up their vulnerable male self-esteem. They have a stable identity in the sense Lichtenstein (1961) described it: an identity core which has undergone relatively little change throughout the various stages and crises of life; it is a kind of basic pattern, a matrix, a red thread running through life as a constant characteristic, forming the foundation for flexibility, adaptation to changing circumstances and creativity. This group makes up about one third of our patients.

Case 8

The 31-year-old university chemist came for therapy of his own accord as he was afraid that his desire to expose himself would jeopardize his social standing.

He is a good-looking, intelligent and apparently discerning person who seems very self-confident, as long as one stays on the intellectual level when conversing with him. He is unsure of himself and inhibited in emotional contact.

He is the fourth of five vicar's children. He describes his father as being a good-natured, helpful and warm-hearted man. His attractive, extrovert mother was the dominating centre of the family and was admired greatly by all, including the patient. Like his siblings, he went to boarding school at 10. He was unhappy to have to leave home and suffered from the separation. However, at school he made good progress and enjoyed learning. He scarcely had any conflicts with his peers, but no close relationships either. His good marks earned him recognition and respect early on.

He was not athletic and did not feel at ease with his body. During puberty he had strong inhibitions about masturbating. He first had a girlfriend at the age of 16; he still remembers this, his one "great love" with sorrow. Although the relationship lasted 3 years, he did not dare make any sexual advances. His mother reacted jealously to his girlfriend, rejected her and warned her son about getting involved with any women at all, of being tied down by marriage and children. The patient blames his mother for this relationship finally breaking up. After this disappointment he turned his entire attention to school and later university. He was very ambitious, dreamt of becoming a famous researcher and was a successful student although his mother had prophesied: "You will never make it." He now lives a somewhat lonely life, only has acquaintances at work and no friends. He is shy and reticent with girls.

One day, when he was a student, he was masturbating in his room when the cleaning lady came in and watched him with interest, or so he says. From then on he developed an initially well-controlled exhibitionistic ritual: he shows his penis from his room when women in the house opposite are looking out of their window. He keeps most of his body hidden. In his phantasy the women watch with interest and enjoy it. He experiences exposing himself as an opportunity to relax and get in touch with himself. This counterbalances the constant pressure he imposes on himself with his high standards. His first sexual contact was with the girl he later married at age 27. Through her he shed his introspective, serious frame of mind and had 2 happy years. A woman was there to care for him, he felt he was in good hands. As she began becoming more independent and drawing away from him, tension developed. He also had erection problems. In the end his wife left him. After the separation his exhibitionist desires which had for the most part disappeared during marriage, were reactivated; they have become so pressing that he is afraid of them getting out of hand.

Psychodynamic Aspects: The patient's central problem is that he is convinced his admired and domineering mother apparently only accepted him as small, dependent and nonsexual. She sent him away when he reached puberty; she could not put up with his interest in other women. She did not even believe he was capable of any intellectual achievements. He was ambitious and managed to be successful at school, university and in his career, but at the price of any spontaneous, emotional or sensual experience of sex. The *symptom* is a compensatory expression of this lack of vivacity and counterbalances his feeling of having been abandoned and left emotionally in a void. In his phantasies he shows off his phallus in a childish ritual finally obtaining the longed-for admiration of and pleasure in his masculinity denied him by his mother.

Therapy see p. 107.

The disturbances in a quarter of our patients were classified as severe or *very severe.* To this group belong patients whose male identity has undergone no or only rudimentary, fragmentary development, whose personality is pervaded by strong and early destructive impulses, whose narcissistic organization is severely impaired and who are more or less incapable of relating to others. These are patients with a borderline structure who have no identifiable stable identity core.

Case 9

We were asked for an expert opinion on this 33-year-old patient who was being prosecuted for rape. After 1 1/2 years in prison he was referred to us for therapy instead of being committed to a psychiatric ward.

He is a large, sturdy man; his arms are tattooed all over. He seems suspicious, taciturn and almost hostile. He emanates a sense of hopelessness and awakens a strong impulse in others to help him.

He was born illegitimately in the German Democratic Republic (GDR). He has never lived with his mother. Nothing is known about the first 5 years of his life. He was sent to a children's home, foster-parents and then another home, ran away frequently and had no real base. In the homes he felt lonely but could hold his own. From the age of 10 on he started secretly adoring girls and idealizing them without daring to approach them. After leaving secondary school his life was again unsettled; while under apprenticeship he moved across to the FRG where he initially wandered around aimlessly. A second attempt at an apprenticeship failed when he was imprisoned for the first time at age 17 for 4 years: as a male prostitute he had been stealing and grabbing women's handbags. Between 1960 and 1976 he spent 11 years in jail for sexual offences. Between sentences he managed to complete a baker's apprenticeship. He liked the job but had to give it up because of a skin eczema. He then withdrew completely from life and vegetated; his life centered on his daydreams and phantasies. Although he has had no real erotic experience at all, in his imagination he has a dream woman with whom he imagines sharing tender embraces and whom he idealizes. He goes to cemeteries and invents conversations with the dead, particularly with children who he wants to comfort.

His *psychosexual development* was marked by a variety of deviant acts around puberty: homosexuality, voyeurism, fetishism and exhibitionism. These urges faded over the years with the gradual emergence of a more distinct sadistic perversion directed against adult women. The perversion became more and more insistent with a pressing uneasiness, excessive masturbation and dramatic phantasies which included murder. He acted extremely violently in the two rapes for which he was prosecuted: he throttled the women and threatened them with a knife.

Psychodynamic Aspects: This patient's personality has been deeply disturbed by early and repeated uprooting. He experiences himself split into good and powerful, evil and powerless fragments; he can only survive by retreating from reality into his phantasies which are a solace for his loneliness and sense of futility, and in which both his desire to be lovingly cared for and his archaic rage can express themselves. The absence of any ability to integrate the good and bad, the splitting in the self-image and lack of impulse control point to a borderline structure. His basic feeling of complete impotence is transformed into destructive omnipotence in the *symptom*, in which his wish for intimacy and shelter suddenly revert into sexualized hatred.

Therapy see p. 126.

When gauging the *severity of the disturbance* the largest group of patients was found to be in *the middle range*. One further criterion we used to assess them was their ability, apart from decompensation in crises, to cope with the problems of everyday life despite their psychopathology.

3.5 Coping Strategies

In discussing diagnosis we began by looking at the significance of the perverse symptoms from three angles: the drive, the narcissistic and the object-libido aspect. Out of this emerged four central problem areas: male identity, the aggression problem, self-image and problems in relating to others. We presented each aspect in turn and a scale for grading how severely disturbed the patients' personalities are.

We should now like to turn to another aspect and ask: which nonperverse defence strategies for the problems mentioned, the anxieties, conflicts and personality defects, can be identified? Ideally this diagnostic process produces an homogenous gestalt of the patient: on the one hand, each underlying problem initiates attempts at sexualized defence which are concentrated in the scenario of the perverse symptom; on the other, this leads to nonperverse defence efforts, which we shall call coping strategies. The same pathology is shown both in the perverse symptom and the coping strategies: they merely represent a different mode of expression.

We understand coping strategies as constantly recurring basic patterns, or typical forms of behaviour which characterize a personality and its way of life. We have already pointed out a similarity with the "interaction strategies" (Wittmann 1981) and "interaction plans" (Grawe and Dziewas 1977) in behaviour therapy.

The concept of the coping strategy becomes clearer if we distinguish it from the psychoanalytic term "defence mechanism"; they involve two different perspectives.

Defence mechanism designates an intrapsychic process in which anxieties resulting from (repressed) instinctual drives or from conflicts arising from them are appeased. This concept is oriented on drives and conflicts and focusses on unconscious processes.

A coping strategy does not refer primarily to intrapsychic processes, but to forms of coping with actual life. The emphasis here is on the type and kind of social interaction. Although coping strategies are also based on anxieties, the anxieties are not attributed to a particular drive and its frustration. As this concept is concerned with what one might call the planning and organization of life, it does not operate on the level of the unconscious, but with preconscious, cognitively accessible mechanisms. This concept is less theoretical and interpretative; instead it contains more elements which can be observed and phenomenologically identified. A coping strategy can be defined as the general compound result of anxieties and defence against them as it is reflected in a person's way of life.

This means that the concept of a coping strategy cannot be subsumed under pathology alone. Certainly, defence mechanisms are only regarded as pathological in the strict sense when they acquire a dominant role over experience and restrict the ego's initiative. In a coping strategy, however, the emphasis is on potential help in organizing a compensatory life-style. The focus is on how a person masters his life in his own characteristic way given certain conditions. In this sense, coping strategies designate both someone's "strengths" and his pathological mechanisms for coping with deficits.

3.5.1 Classifying Coping Strategies Using Factor Analysis

A brief reminder of our procedure so far: first, we roughly assessed 32 patient histories and outlined the strategies which we considered typical for each patient. This produced a variety of initially uncorrelated typical behaviour patterns. From these we inductively formed categories, i.e. we picked out the strategies mentioned most frequently in our rough assessment. After classifying all 86 patients using these categories, 33 strategies were factor analysed to identify typical structures. When using the term coping strategies below we are speaking on the factor level and not on the level of individual strategies.

Factor analysis[2] resulted in a ten-factor solution which explained 75% of the total variance. To mark the factors, factor loadings of $\geqq 0.40$ were used. The factors are listed in order of significance according to the degree of variance they explain.

1. *"Avoiding intimacy" vs. "search for dependency in relationships"* (23.2% of total variance; 34.3% of explained variance)
Categories
- Avoiding commitment in relationships (0.75)
- Constant withdrawal (0.66)
- Opposition (0.53)
- Withholding feelings (0.50)
- Childlike dependency/clinging (-0.81)
- Dependency in relationships (-0.78)
- Passive compliance/masochistic submission (-0.65)

2. *"Manipulative, indirect aggression"* (10.5% of total variance; 14.5% of explained variance)
Categories
- Covert aggression to achieve ends (0.79)
- Projecting aggressive impulses (0.68)
- Manipulating/functionalizing (0.66)
- Delegating responsibility (0.57)
- Denigrating others (0.47)

3. *"Escape into ideal phantasy world"* (9.4% of total variance; 12.8% of explained variance)
Categories
- Escape into phantasy/dream world (0.65)
- Altruism (0.62)
- Idealization (0.59)
- Escape into phantasized ideal relationship (0.58)

4. *"Overt aggression and opposition"* vs. "harmonization" (7.1% of total variance; 9.4% of explained variance)
Categories
- Overt aggression/self-assertion (0.79)
- Demonstrating independence/stereotype manliness (0.64)
- Antagonistic behaviour (0.64)
- Defiance (0.53)
- Denigrating others (0.43)
- Playing down problems/harmonization (– 0.40)

5. *"Autoaggression"* (5.8% of total variance; 7.2% of explained variance)
Categories
- Presenting oneself in a negative light (making oneself unlovable, unattractive) (0.68)
- Hostility directed inwards/ self-sabotage (0.64)

6. *"Hyperactivity"* (5.2% of total variance 6.2% of explained variance)
Categories
- Hyperactivity/keeping busy (0.62)

7. *"Withdrawal from relationships" vs. "indiscriminate relationships"* (4% of total variance; 4.5% of explained variance)
Categories

[2] Principal axis factor analysis; number of extracted factors according to the criterion eigenvalue > 1; varimax rotation. We are aware of the problems involved in factor analysis, particularly regarding the level of measurement for our data; we nevertheless regard it as fruitful as a heuristic method.

- Social isolation (0.81)
- Narcissistic withdrawal (0.71)
- Seeking safety in numbers (- 0.50)

8. "Compensating via achievement and adaptation" (3.9% of total variance; 4.3% of explained variance)
Categories
- Exaggerating achievement/intellectuality/success/perfection (0.64)
- Compulsive rigidity (0.63)
- Acting roles/hiding behind masks (0.49)

9. "Invoking sympathy with childlike behaviour" (3.3% of total variance; 3.5% of explained variance)
Category
- Demonstrating harmlessness/helplessness/childishness (0.80)

10. "Insisting on attention" (3.2% of total variance; 3.4% of explained variance)
Category
- Theatrical behaviour/courting admiration (0.78)

In the following these factors will be discussed statistically as *new characteristics* and descriptively as *coping strategies*. Factors 6, 9 and 10 contain only one variable. There is therefore no point in interpreting these variables on the factor level. Factor 6 (variable: "hyperactivitiy") designates a defence strategy in which hectic activity is employed mainly as a defence against depression. Factor 9 ("invoking sympathy with childlike behaviour") designates a behaviour pattern which is typified by denying any hostile impulses and shying away from conflicts. Factor 10 ("insisting on attention") is a strategy for compensating a negative self-image. Particularly as these three characteristics do not load in other factors, they should be treated as important separate strategies. This leaves seven factors.

Table 5. Frequency of pronounced coping strategies observed

Coping strategies	n	Pronounced %	Pronounced %	Coping strategies 2nd factor pole
1. Avoiding intimacy vs. search for dependency	61	28	26	Search for dependency in relationships
2. Manipulative indirect aggression	58	34	-	-
3. Escape into phantasized ideal world	57	25	-	-
4. Overt aggression and opposition	60	20	15	Harmonization
5. Autoaggression	53	36	-	-
6. Withdrawal from relationships	62	39	5	Indiscriminate relationships
7. Compensating via achievement and adaptation	60	18	-	-

In order to assess the relevance of the coping strategies, the distribution of values of each strategy was translated back into our usual classification nonexistent, slight and pronounced. In Table 5 we have listed how often a coping strategy was observed *in pronounced form*. We have skipped the categories slight and nonexistent in order to make the table more readable and also because most of the strategies are fairly common and are behaviour patterns reaching well into healthy areas. A coping strategy is only psychodiagnostically important if it is pronounced and thus a key theme.

We also took the correlations between the coping strategies into account (see Table 6).

Table 6. Coping strategies. Correlations (r ≧0.30)

Coping strategies	1	2	3	4	5	6	7
1. Avoiding intimacy vs. search for dependency							
2. Manipulative indirect aggression	0.45						
3. Escape into phantasized ideal world							
4. Overt aggression and opposition vs. harmonization	0.60	0.55					
5. Autoaggression							
6. Withdrawal from relationships vs. indiscriminate relationships			0.41		0.37		
7. Compensating via achievement and adaptation							

Tables 5 and 6 taken together produce the following picture: Factor 1, "Avoiding intimacy" vs. "search for dependency in relationships", has key significance: most variables are subsumed under it, more than half the patients showed high values on the negative or positive pole; hardly any patients were neutral. The two factors involving aggressive strategies directed outwards (factors 2 and 4) are closely associated with factor 1: the stronger and more frequently "avoiding intimacy" appears, the more frequent use is made of aggressive strategies directed against others. "Manipulative, indirect aggression" (factor 2) plays a larger role than "overt aggression" (factor 4) and they correlate strongly. Strategies involving withdrawal are relatively independent of factor 1: "withdrawal from relationships" (factor 7) and "escape into phantasized ideal world" (factor 3); these two factors show a marked correlation. "Autoaggression" (factor 5) is relatively independent of the other strategies, particularly of those with outwardly directed aggression. The strategy "compensating via achievement and adaptation" (factor 8) is independent of all the others.

3.5.2 Typical Coping Strategies (Factor Interpretation)

In our interpretation of the separate factors illustrated by case histories below one should take the following into account: a patient's coping strategies are never characterized by *one* factor *alone*, not even by the factor used to describe the patient. The patients' histories also clearly show that their specific behaviour patterns only take shape as a bundle of factors.

Moreover, a single factor never characterizes a particular intensity of disorder or a specific pathology. The psychodynamic background and stabilizing function of the coping strategies reflected in the factors can vary considerably in quality - depending on each patient's structure and problem. It is important to remember this to avoid mistaking the factors for stereotype patterns or labels.

Factor 1: Avoiding Intimacy vs. Search for Dependency in Relationships

This factor has two poles:

a) In contrast to factor 7 ("withdrawal from relationships"), the pole "avoiding intimacy" does not mean complete isolation, but rather a narrower and more restricted social context in which a person can maintain an inner distance. Close emotional relationships with others are avoided, life takes place in a kind of recess to which one can withdraw, frequently with the feeling of being an outsider. This coping strategy was pronounced in a quarter of the patients. No significant correlation with the kind of offence and the intensity of the deviancy was found. In terms of their basic problem, patients with a tendency towards illusions of grandeur in their self-image ($p < 1\%$), considerable aggression potential ($p < 1\%$) and less ability to form relationships ($p < 1\%$) tend particularly to adopt this coping strategy. Factor 1 is also linked to nonsexual criminality ($p < 1\%$), poorer social integration ($p < 1\%$) and a strong tendency to sexualize relationships ($p < 1\%$). The link with aggression seems to be important: avoiding intimacy also seems to have the function of protecting oneself and others from one's own aggressive impulses.

In general terms this strategy is an attempt to cope usually observed in more severely disturbed patients who are poorly integrated socially and whose narcissistic organization and ability to relate to others are impaired.

b) The second pole is the *search for dependency in relationships*. It is characterized by a tendency to comply, submit, to lean on and cling to others in a childish way. This strategy was pronounced in a quarter of the patients. No significant correlations with the kind of offence or intensity of the deviancy were found here either, although aspects of their basic problem were involved: patients with a strongly negative self-image ($p < 5\%$) and a childish relationship structure ($p < 1\%$) tend more towards this behaviour pattern. The psychic stabilization provided by this strategy is greater than in "avoiding intimacy" as the strategy is found mostly in depressive, dependent patients who are less severely disturbed and are more likely to find refuge in relationships which stabilize them.

We identified the coping strategy outlined by factor 1 in the following case history (with both poles).

Case 10

The long prison sentence of this 43-year-old patient was suspended on the condition that he seek therapy. He had been convicted before for exhibitionism and in recent years for burglaries which were closely linked to a voyeuristic perversion.

He is small, sturdy in stature and comes to sessions exhausted and still in his working clothes. He feels guilty, is contrite, mistrustful, taciturn and resigned. When speaking of himself he always seems to be asking for pardon. His submissiveness makes it difficult to develop a more animated relationship to him.

The dominating figure in his life has always been his mother. Although almost completely blind, she has kept the family together and earned their living. He has always admired her, felt obliged to do all he could for her and constantly felt guilty for not coming up to her expectations. He has never quite been able to get away from her although he has often felt very restricted by her. His father returned from the war as a semicripple. He played a minor role in the family, drank and shirked all responsibility. The patient was often sent to bring him back from the bar. He was his mother's problem child, was ill much more often than his younger sister and developed behavioural disorders such as enuresis and encopresis.

After leaving elementary school he completed a plumber's apprenticeship; work, achievement and success are decisive aspects in his life. He wanted to prove to his mother that he was capable of something. He was respected at work, was always on call and was unable to say no, but had no friends or private relationships.

He remembers a scene from childhood in which his mother was raped by Russian soldiers while he looked on helplessly. In puberty he began spying on his mother and sister and, soon after, neighbouring women and girls when they were undressing. His first steady relationship at 19 was with his later wife who suffered from epilepsy. At his mother's request they came to live with her. Conflicts soon arose as he was inwardly on his mother's side and constantly compared his wife with her. He had an unerotic relationship to his wife; they divorced after 2 years of marriage. He stayed with his mother. He very soon entered into another marriage which ran along the same lines: the couple lived with his mother who constantly interfered in the relationship. Marital sexuality was unsatisfying; he had erection dysfunctions and was only potent during his regular brothel visits. He felt inferior to his wife and felt she gave him the cold shoulder. This was when he exposed himself to women for the first time. At 25 the voyeuristic perversion set in, took up a great deal of his attention and became almost his only interest outside work. He was convicted several times as a result. He gradually started forcing his way into women's apartments where he rummaged for objects which he then pocketed. Matters worsened when he began pulling the bedding off sleeping women and girls; he always fled the moment they woke up. He was also fascinated by the excitement inherent in the situation and the risk of being discovered. When he began losing all control over the perverse impulses, he asked his wife to pick him up from work. This reminds one of his helpless, weak father who always had to be picked up from the bars. During a lengthy imprisonment his wife divorced him. After his release, his mother died. He then immediately remarried his first wife. The marriage is as problematic as ever. He feels inferior and under her thumb. He likes being cared for by her like a little boy and feels obliged to her. They have little in common with each other. In the relationships to his two wives, who are the only points of contact in his loneliness, a pattern recurs which was also typical of the mother-son relationship: while being dependent, subordinating himself and always making an effort to come up to all expectations, he is also emotionally reserved, withdraws and is unable to establish a really intimate relationship (impotence, lack of erotic interest).

Psychodynamic Aspects: This patient's main problem is that he has failed to separate from his mother, without ever having come really close to her emotionally because she expected too much of him, left him to his own devices and expected him to be self-sufficient too early on – the son was the only "man" in the family in view of his often absent, weak father. The patient experiences himself as defenceless and dependent when relating to women. The ensuing aggression is, on the one hand, coped with autodestructively (constant guilt feelings, depressive moods, submissiveness and self-destructive acting out) and, on the other, emerges in the *symptom*. It has the function of giving him a feeling of superiority and potency and of overcoming his sense of powerlessness with women by letting him get close to them in a situation where they cannot defend themselves. Forcing his way into others' apartments and taking away objects is linked with the exhilaration of a risk he constantly has to face; symbolically he attacks and robs the women of their power. The symptom is an escape from the prison of his relationship which can nevertheless be maintained, as it is quite separate from the symptom.

Therapy see p. 111.

Factor 2: "Manipulative, Indirect Aggression"

Factor 2 is a behaviour pattern characterized by diffuse aggressive impulses or defence against them: responsibility is delegated, aggressive impulses are projected outwards in a paranoid manner. The subject builds up his own self-esteem by running down others. Given their inability to feel empathy, these patients usually see relationships as a means of satisfying their own needs; they functionalize and manipulate other people. This coping strategy was pronounced in one third of our patients. There is a significant correlation with sexually aggressive symptoms ($p<1\%$) and severe deviancy ($p<5\%$). In terms of their basic problem, patients in this group are mostly severely disturbed ($p<5\%$), have a fragmentary male identity ($p<1\%$), have illusions of grandeur ($p<1\%$), a greater aggression potential ($p<1\%$), little control over their aggressive impulses ($p<1\%$), little ability to relate to others ($p<1\%$), few social contacts ($p<1\%$), and have a history of nonsexual criminality ($p<1\%$) and alcoholism ($p<5\%$).

Generally speaking, this attempt to cope is found in severely disturbed patients without social ties who maintain a hostile, paranoid distance to those around them. Being closed off inside themselves, they are scarcely capable of anything else but using other people; this naturally makes therapy with them difficult.

The following patient showed elements of this factor.

Case 11

The patient (28 years old) was referred to us by a counselling centre because he was depressive and suicidal, had failed to regain a foothold after the death of his mother a year earlier and was distressed by homosexual pedophile desires. Court proceedings began after therapy had started.

He looks untidy and distinctly older than he really is. He is very unresponsive, suspicious and awkward and makes a bizarre, eccentric impression. He seems partly helplessly depressive, partly reproachful and accusing.

He was born illegitimately in Romania where he first grew up with his mother and his (3 years) older brother. He describes his mother as being a strict, cold, energetic and dominating woman who gave him a great deal of attention as he was the weak and ailing problem child.

His brother was much more robust and independent and the patient still maintains a shy, respectful distance to him today. His upbringing was strictly religious and still influences him. Despite his close ties to his mother he received little comfort from her; she was not very loving, regimented, restricted and punished him. At the age of 8 he, his mother and his brother moved to the FRG. Adapting was difficult for him. He had problems at school because of the language, was teased and frequently beaten up by the others. He was afraid of other children and was unable to defend himself. After leaving secondary school he took various jobs as an unskilled labourer. He reacted to his frequent dismissals with angry accusations. He lived with his mother until he was 24. He is very isolated, has hardly any social contacts, takes no pleasure in life and lets himself drift. His only comfort is in phantasizing about his old home. He lives under the delusion that the resettlement was the only cause of his misfortune; everything would be fine if he were to go back. Full of accusations, he makes his environment responsible for his misery. His mother's death represented a hiatus in his life; he has been aware of his lack of roots ever since; everything seems senseless and without any perspective. Sexuality has been a problem for him right from the start. Around puberty he already felt sexually attracted to children of both sexes, especially to small boys. This triggered strong moral qualms which led to his first suicide attempt. He has great difficulty talking about these problems. He hints at having had sexual contact with boys now and again. He is preoccupied by sexual phantasies of bathing with boys, lathering, drying and spoiling them.

He generally avoids entering into relationships and has hardly any contact to women. He first had a girlfriend at the age of 20, but he did not dare to approach her physically. He sensed that she expected more of him, but was afraid of failing. When she finally left him he again tried to commit suicide.

When his mother died he joined up with an older woman, a kind of mother-substitute, who has 2 sons aged 9 and 12. He moved in with her, lets her take care of him but constantly complains about the cramped quarters. When they quarrel he threatens to kill himself. This relationship is the first time he has had any heterosexual contact although he does not reach orgasm, just as in the pedophile contacts. Consequently he tends more and more to withdraw, but cannot understand his partner's disappointment. The two boys are obviously the real attraction for him. He sees fatherly love as a right to physical affection to which he reproachfully lays claim.

Psychodynamic Aspects: Psychogenetically the decisive point seems to be that the patient always lived in close proximity to and within the control and grasp of his mother, without feeling sheltered or cared for by her. Lacking any other identification figure, he has remained highly dependent, is not self-sufficient and has been unable to develop his own identity. Particularly since his mother's death he has led a lonely and rootless life like a lost child in an environment felt to be hostile and takes refuge in infantile dreams of a better world. He is extremely envious and resentful; through lack of empathy, he can only relate to others as a source of care. When his unquenchable oral claims to be looked after are not satisfied, he either acts out autodestructive tendencies (suicide attempts) or, by projecting his aggressive impulses, sees himself as the victim of a hostile environment which gives him the right to insist on being taken care of without assuming any responsibility for himself. The *symptom* is the attempt to establish a perfect union with the mother through projective identification; he can experience himself both as mother and child by sexualizing his pregenital desires in a kind of acting out by swapping roles. All his emotional energy and vivacity seem to sucked up into the world of his perversion.

Therapy see p. 96.

Factor 3: "Escape into a Phantasized Ideal World"

Factor 3 describes a striking coping strategy which seems to be an isolated phenomenon and to have few links with other characteristics. It is pronounced in a quarter of the patients and is characterized by withdrawal, denial of aggression and escape from a reality patients experience as frightening and overtaxing into an ideal phantasy world - a coping strategy which is found above all in immature and childish ($p < 1\%$), depressive ($p < 1\%$) and idealizing, dreamy and harmonizing patients, often combined with pedophile symptoms ($p < 1\%$). The following case history is a good example.

Case 12

The 30-year-old patient was not under pressure from criminal proceedings, but he was afraid of getting into trouble with the law on account of his homosexual, pedophile tendencies.

He is a slender, pale, youthful looking patient who appears clumsy and taciturn. Making contact is difficult.

He is the eldest son of an attorney. His sister and brothers were born in rapid succession after him. His first brother (-1 years) was better adapted to life and was the parents' pet. His sister (-2) moved away from home fairly early. His mentally handicapped youngest brother (-4) made great demands on the parents. The patient had a difficult relationship to his father who was strict, autocratic and had high expectations of his eldest son. Whenever the latter failed to fulfill them, he was punished. The patient still feels constantly under pressure today from his father's demands on him. He rejects his father but unconsciously compares himself with him and still feels inferior to him. He describes his mother as being cold and dismissive: his longing for affection fell on deaf ears. In the family he felt isolated and lonely. He stayed at secondary school until the final school examination. He was just as much a loner among his peers, never had friends, and was awkward and inhibited. His interests focussed on activities which allowed him to be on his own. He played the harpsichord, read a lot, indulged in daydreams of living a self-sufficient life in unspoilt nature and burying himself in ancient manuscripts. He studied archaeology and then worked in a museum.

Essentially he has been a pedophile homosexual since puberty. With women he feels extremely anxious and inferior and maintains a timid distance. He had not had any heterosexual experiences when therapy began. Anything to do with his body makes him inhibited and embarrassed. He was in his early twenties when he became aware of his homosexual, pedophile desires. At a boys' choir concert he had phantasies in which he adored boys and was fascinated by their "angelic" appearance. More out of curiosity he contacted a young homosexual man through an advertisement and later had several encounters with male prostitutes. He is interested in adolescent boys; he makes friends with them and enthuses about these meetings. Genital sex in these relationships, as in his phantasies, is of little importance. He wants friendship and affection; he looks after them when they are not well and usually chooses boys who are social outcasts. Otherwise he devotes his life entirely to himself, spends his time on music and his daydreams, suffers from feelings of loneliness, emptiness, meaninglessness and depression; he feels inferior and unfulfilled; his basic feeling in life is one of anxiety.

Psychodynamic Aspects: In the threatening and frightening shadow of this father, the patient had, as it were, no light to nourish his growth and maturation. His mother, probably overstrained by so many children, was a cold woman who gave him scarcely any firm ground to strike root. Any attention he received tended to be in the form of criticism. Just as his parents never accepted him for what he was, he too was unable to accept himself. Being the eldest he was seldom allowed to be a child and had to try to meet demands made on him which he could not satisfy. His personality is marked by a constant feeling of being put under pressure by excessive demands. He experiences reality as loveless and exacting and avoids it by withdrawing as a lone wolf into a self-sufficient, consoling, but objectless dream world. In the *symptom,* his wishes are fulfilled through identification: by fulfilling the desires of (usually) destitute boys for care and shelter - unfulfilled in himself - he fuses with a happier alter ego. In his pedophile relationships he loses the feeling of loneliness, insecurity and inner emptiness, and momentarily feels comforted and alive.

Therapy see p. 109.

Factor 4: "Overt Aggression and Opposition" vs. "Harmonization"

Factor 4 has two poles:

a) "Overt aggression and opposition": as with factor 2, aggression is the main element in this coping strategy. Here, however, it is used offensively and is not indirect and hidden as in factor 2. It involves confrontation, a demonstration of strength and autonomy. This coping strategy was pronounced in one fifth of the patients. There were significant correlations with aggressive sexual symptoms ($p<5\%$), pronounced deviancy ($p<5\%$), grandiose ideas about the self ($p<1\%$), a large aggression potential ($p<1\%$), poor control over aggressive impulses ($p<1\%$), little ability to relate to others ($p<1\%$), and also with nonsexual criminality ($p<1\%$) and poor social integration ($p<5\%$).

The typical variables of this pole are those associated with clearly defined adult masculinity (assertion, intimidating behaviour). When our patients used this behaviour pattern as a coping strategy it frequently had a contraphobic function: it involved progressive reactions in the sense of resorting to counter-attack in order to conceal their general vulnerability and underlying feelings of weakness. These patients often regard themselves as lone wolves (see Case 17).

b) The *second pole* is marked only by the category "minimalizing conflicts, harmonization" which only has a load of 0.40, so we do not believe it is worth interpreting this category on the factor level. As it crops up frequently as a variable, however, we regard it as a significant independent strategy. It is found in Cases 6, 12, 14 and 15.

Factor 5: "Autoaggression"

The fifth factor again designates a coping strategy in which aggression plays the main role; however, in this case it is directed neither covertly nor overtly outwards but at the patient's own person. Autoaggression was very pronounced in one third of the patients. The high incidence of this factor gives some indication of the patients' obstacles in accepting themselves. These vary from strict scruples, a damaging tendency to sabotage anything constructive they try to do, to deep hatred and autodestructive behaviour patterns. These patients were assessed as severely disturbed ($p<5\%$), the symptom was becoming more severe ($p<5\%$); they had an extremely negative self-image ($p<1\%$), a generally depressive view on life ($p<1\%$), severe problems with relationships ($p<1\%$) and were socially isolated ($p<5\%$). Aspects of this factor can be found in Cases 3, 4, 10 and 11.

Factor 6: "Withdrawal from Relationships" vs. "Indiscriminate Relationships"

This factor also has two poles:

a) "Withdrawal from relationships": this pole is associated with "avoiding intimacy" in factor 1. Social and emotional withdrawal are more total and uncompromising in this coping strategy. Relationships are not just kept at an impersonal level but are avoided altogether. The tendency here is to withdraw into isolation and loneliness, into a life by oneself. About two fifths of the patients used this coping strategy in a pronounced form. They were more often severely disturbed ($p<5\%$), had a frail male identity ($p<5\%$), a negative self-image ($p<5\%$), a generally depressive view on life ($p<5\%$), less ability to relate to others ($p<1\%$) and were hardly integrated in society ($p<1\%$). Some aspects of this coping strategy can be seen in the following case history.

Case 13

The 36-year-old patient, who had been sentenced several times for indecent exposure to ado lescent boys, made intensive efforts to find therapy and was prepared to travel long distances

He is a small, wiry man who looks much younger than he is and seems altogether very tense, reticent and uneasy. He has a marked tendency to rationalize and evade emotions.

He grew up in chaotic surroundings. His mother, a part-time prostitute, gave birth to him illegitimately. He does not know his father. Until the age of 5 he lived with his grandmothe who spoilt him materially but gave him little affection. He describes her as being a woman with strict principles, quite different from his mother who then took him back. She was very fickle, married quickly three times in succession and had six more children in the process. Th family lived in cramped conditions, the mother was often away and neglected the children The patient also had little contact to his brothers and sisters. He withdrew into himself earl on and felt lonely. When his mother and grandmother died he hardly grieved. He took to pet ty theft early on which ended in him being committed to a home where he stayed until leaving school. He got on well, was not homesick, but had scarcely any contact to other children. A school he was an enthusiastic pupil, his marks were good and he greatly enjoyed anything tha had to do with intellect and achievement. He then began a mechanic's apprenticeship and lived in an apprentices' home. He had broken off all ties with his family. During this period h began regularly breaking into cars. Similar to his urge to expose himself, this developed out o a feeling of inner emptiness combined with the exhilaration and intoxication of speedin around in the stolen cars. At age 17 he was repeatedly sentenced and spent a total of 11 year in jail. In prison he continued his education and gained a diploma in programming. The las time he was discharged was 3 years prior to therapy. He no longer breaks into cars, lives alon in a small apartment, has a good position in his profession and gets on well with others a work on a formal level. He only gets into a heated argument "once a year" when he has to many feelings bottled up. His colleagues concede him this right. He has lofty and unrealisti notions about friendship and does not want to come out of his isolation. He has no intimat relationships for fear of being disappointed and rejected.

Sexuality has always played a comforting role. He has had scarcely any erotic experience: He slept with a girlfriend for the first time at age 27. They stayed together for 2 years and ha a son; however, a close emotional bond apparently did not develop. After she left him he onl had sporadic, fleeting contacts to women. He has no potency problems ("at least that works" He has a deep desire to feel safe which he does not dare show.

The problem of indecent exposure has existed since puberty and became more pressing a the symptom of breaking into cars lost its importance. The two symptoms are similar in signif icance and function. He exposes his penis mostly to boys, acting very reticently and passively When the boys see him he pretends they surprised him. Occasionally these situations lead t sexual acts with them; once a slightly longer erotic relationship developed. He is fascinated b boys who act with ease and aplomb. He disapproves of his need to expose himself, is ashame of himself and feels contemptible as a result.

Psychodynamic Aspects: His chaotic childhood and adolescence, with the frequent uprooting and the complete lack of loving attention to his needs as a child, forced this patient early on t take charge of his life himself. The lack of any good inner objects led to withdrawal and mis trust and prevented him from approaching other people emotionally or becoming intimat with anyone. A progressive defence, in which his intellectual inquisitiveness, his ability and his ambition play an important role, enable him to maintain his self-esteem. In the perverse *symptom* the patient, by identifying with the boys who represent a vivacious counterpart to himself, can break out of the barrenness of his unemotional world. Not only is a narcisstic exhilaration involved, as in the earlier symptom of breaking into cars, but also a shy attempt at courting attention and admiration to help him escape from his loneliness.

Therapy see p. 95.

Factor 7: "Compensating via Achievement and Adaptation"

This factor is an important and characteristic coping strategy observed in a pronounced form in one fifth of the patients. The strategy is found frequently in patients who try to incorporate a high degree of social desirability into their way of life, who derive their self-esteem from being a success, and adapt their life to the constant fulfillment of norms and expectations. This goes hand in hand with a certain rigidity; these patients are not very self-reliant, rarely spontaneous and seem to disappear, as it were, in the role they embody. Consequently, their offences form a crass contrast to the decent face they present to the world. This factor is found significantly more often in patients who were assessed as being less disturbed ($p < 1\%$). The following case history is a good example.

Case 14

The 42-year-old patient had been convicted previously several times for indecent exposure to women and came to therapy because prosecution was again pending.

He is a small, lively, corpulent man with a rosy face and a humble attitude; he puts on an assiduous air and tries to make a good impression. It is difficult to introduce a more personal note into the conventional atmosphere of therapy sessions.

He comes from a well-ordered background. Little was found out about his relationship to his parents. He describes himself as having been a soft, fearful "mother's boy" who was rarely angry, found making contact difficult, stuttered and was afraid of the dark. Since puberty he has had an acute adiposis which he regards as an added handicap. In his work he is ambitious and conscientious; he rose from unskilled worker to warehouseman. Since 1969 he has been a self-employed real estate agent and his business is flourishing.

One outstanding childhood memory is a scene in which his hands were tied because he had been playing with his genitals; his parents threatened to put him in a home. He remembers having to take care of his younger, delicate sister a great deal and was always admonished to treat her with care. He was shy towards girls; he was, and still is, a lone wolf. During sporadic brothel visits he had potency problems. After having built up his business and means of existence, he met his wife through an advertisement at the age of 32. He married because it was simply "the thing to do", but it was not a love affair. The partners have got used to each other, their life together has neither ups nor downs. Sexuality plays no major role. From the very start, neither felt the other was particularly attractive physically. In the course of the marriage his wife developed eczema and began to drink, which appears to have been an opportunity he welcomed to give up any kind of physical intimacy.

His exhibitionist problem has existed since puberty. He is deeply ashamed of it as it is completely irreconcilable with his idea of middle-class decency. Here, too, he tries to behave "correctly"; he asks women to give him permission to show himself to them. In his phantasies he longs for them to be amused by his genitals and to jeer at him.

Psychodynamic Aspects: As the patient recounts little about himself it is difficult to reconstruct his development. However, everything seems to suggest that home life was dominated by an "anal" atmosphere: getting on in life, maintaining appearances, renouncing drives and sup pressing anger, which forced him into a straitjacket which left no room for emotionality, liveli ness and spontaneity. The suppressed anger is shown in the destructive elements which per vade his phantasies about sexuality and masculinity. The patient lives in a kind of prison o conventions in which only achievement carries any positive weight. The *symptom* is the ex pression of his protest against these restrictions, although the phantasies of being ridiculed b: women immediately wipe out the pleasure of experiencing his masculinity and potency. Iı this way he reassures himself that his phallus is harmless and not dangerous. His system o conventions is left untouched by this masochistic submission.

Therapy see p. 108.

3.6 Assigning Patients to Groups (Cluster Analysis)

So far we have broken down the overall problem into its various aspects an(described them in turn. Multiple overlapping was inevitable: the meaning of ; perverse symptom and the coping strategies reflect the basic problem, and th(basic problem is expressed by the symptom and coping strategies. Each o these aspects is multilayered and complex. A tightly spun web emerges whicl might seem intricate and confusing. Nonetheless, we believe it makes sense t(describe each individual aspect in turn; to avoid an oversimplified analysis it i: worth taking the trouble to examine the many facets involved.

In the previous chapters we repeatedly pointed out how important it is t(have a *synoptic overview*. In this final diagnostic chapter we should like to la: out possible guidelines for achieving such an overview. Using cluster analysi we examined how many patient groups could be found which can be usefull: interpreted. Cluster analysis produced five groups, of which four correspondec closely with our clinical observations. They differ markedly from one anothei are distinctly separate and can be clearly described both on the phenomenolog ical and the psychodynamic level. We were confirmed here in our repeated ref erence to the great heterogeneity of these patients. The cluster analysis result should, however, be interpreted with one reservation: cluster analysis is a rela tively crude method on a highly abstract level. The groups represent no mor(than a rough orientation and classification guide and should not be overinter preted as a fixed set of types. With this in mind, we have placed the cluste analysis results at the end of the section on diagnosis, and not at the beginning as we did not want to suggest they have a significance they in fact do not merit

We employed two cluster analysis methods based on different principles of cluster identifica tion: the one hierarchic/agglomerative and the other ipsative.[3] We included 14 variables w considered important. The variables were dichotomized.

The following criteria determined our *selection of variables*: we were mainly concerned witl finding *groupings* within the "basic problem". Variables in the significance of a perverse symp tom and in the coping strategies were therefore not included. We determined the correlatioı with these variables statistically. For the sake of clarity we confined ourselves to relatively fe\

[3] We made use of Wishart's cluster analysis program packet.

variables and chose those which were not only significant but also could be dichotomized in a meaningful way.

The following variables were used:

1. *Assessment of severity of personality pathology.*
2. *Variables in the basic problem* as regards *masculinity problems,* assessment of "male identity" could not be reasonably dichotomized. This aspect is only repesented by the variable "potency disorders". *Aggression problems* were covered by the variables "aggression potential" and "aggression control". The *narcissistic aspect* is contained in "self-image", "depressive view on life" and "suicidal tendencies". Finally, "intimacy problems" are covered by "ability to relate to others".
3. *Psychic symptom formation.* The variables "psychosomatic disorders", "alcoholism" and nonsexual "criminality" were selected.
4. Two variables on *sexual deviancy* were included: "intensity of deviancy" and "use of violence in offences".
5. Our overall *parameter for stability* was "social integration".

After identifying the groups, the characteristics were "undichotomized" so as to describe them in detail. At first 47 patients, for whom we had data for all 14 characteristics, were included in the cluster analysis. After the groups had been identified, 13 additional patients were assigned to the groups for whom data were missing in only one of the 14 characteristics; thus, a total of 60 of 86 patients were included.

To identify interpretable groups we first looked at the growth in heterogeneity of clusters in both methods while the number of clusters decreased. While taking into account undersized groups, the result was that the best solutions were the three, four or five clusters. These three solutions were considered in both methods. The results showed that both methods and all the solutions were always evident in two clusters, but were most pronounced in the five-cluster solutions. We therefore employed a five-cluster solution. To find out whether the hierarchical or ipsative cluster solution should be selected, we compared the other three clusters in both methods.

Distinct similarities were found between the groups in both methods; the hierarchical method, however, produced the most pronounced group in terms of characteristic and patient breakdown, which is why we chose this method. Table 7 illustrates the separate clusters.

Below we shall describe the individual clusters.

3.6.1 Psychically Relatively Stable, Socially Integrated Patients (Cluster 1)

In the *description of variables* (see Table 7) of this cluster these patients are assessed as being the most stable and least pathological. Their ability to enter into relationships is only slightly impaired; their self-image is usually consistent without any grandiose aspects. They are generally not depressive. Pronounced inhibition of aggression is characteristic: they are not noticeably aggressive and their aggression is kept under firm control. These patients are generally socially and professionally integrated. They neither show any signs of socially undesirable symptoms such as criminality or alcoholism, nor any psychosomatic symptoms or tendency towards suicide. Their deviancy is not insistent nor does it become progressively more severe; in some cases the deviancy is a rare reaction to crises. The sexual offences committed by these patients are almost always

Table 7. The results of cluster analysis

	Group 1 (n = 13)	Group 2 (n = 13)	Group 3 (n = 7)	Group 4 (n = 12)	Group 5 (n = 15)
Severity of personality pathology	Almost always slight	Almost always slight or medium	Almost always slight or medium	Not uniform	Always medium or strong
Potency dysfunctions	Not uniform	Always present	Not uniform	None or only slight	Not uniform often severe
Aggression potential	Almost always slight	Not uniform	Almost always medium or strong	Almost always medium or strong	Almost always strong
Aggression control	Always present	Not uniform	Almost always low	Not uniform	Almost always low
Self-image	Almost always self-acceptance	Almost always negative self-concept	Not uniform	Not uniform	Not uniform, mostly illusions of grandeur
Depressive view on life	Almost never	Almost always pronounced	Always none or only slight	Always none or only slight	Not uniform
Suicidal tendencies	Almost never	Not uniform	Almost never	Not uniform	Not uniform
Ability to relate to others	As a rule limited but not always	Not uniform	Always limited	Always limited or severely disturbed	Almost always severely disturbed
Psychosomatic disorders	Almost never	Not uniform	Almost always	Almost never	Not uniform
Alcoholism	Almost never	Not uniform	Always present	Not uniform	Not uniform
Criminality	Never	Almost never	Always present	Not uniform	Almost always present
Intensity of deviancy	As a rule firmly established, partly established deviation	Almost always firmly established, partly increasing severity	Almost always firmly established, no increasing severity	Always firmly established, no increasing severity	Almost always increasing in severity
Violence in offence	Mostly none	Mostly none, present in part	Not uniform	None	Almost always present
Social integration	Always good or medium	Almost always medium	Almost always medium, partly good	Not uniform	Always poor

nonviolent. This group consists almost entirely of patients who expose their genitals to women and children; other offences are scarcely encountered. This does not mean, however, that exhibitionism is restricted to this group alone. The correlation with coping strategies in this cluster shows that these patients prefer autoaggressive and withdrawal strategies and tend towards "compensating via achievement and adaptation".

The variables described are merely an orientation guide; they are cornerstones, but do not represent the entire building. We can draw on our discussions in previous chapters to fill in the gaps and erect a kind of prototype gestalt.

These patients' psychic structure is less severely disturbed; they have an identity with a clearly contoured personality core which helps them to live inconspicuously in society, be successful at work and adapt well - at least superficially - to reality's requirements. Their coping strategies underline more their strengths than the pathological mechanisms. Although they are capable of relating to others, stability is secured only by choosing relationships in which they take the dependent role and tie themselves to domineering, strict women. The harmony of such partnerships is guaranteed by the patients' inability to assert themselves in a manly way, their behaviour in general being almost exclusively nonaggressive. They derive recognition and admiration from their achievements but conform closely to the expectations of their environment. The relatively close correlation found between this group and the meaning behind the symptom "act of defiance" ($C = 0.47$) indicates that the symptom's function is to liberate the patient in particular from the restrictions impeding his phallic-narcissistic development and to make him feel independent and potent.

The perverse symptom, mainly exhibitionism, is not the expression of a fixed perversion but of a perverse reaction (see Sect. 3.2.1). It is a momentary breakout, a protest against being locked in and dependent. The symptom gives the patient a sense of being alive and strong which serves temporarily to restore or replenish his confidence in his maleness in situations of crisis and frustration when his compensation mechanisms prove inadequate. The symptom is circumscribed and can be isolated, contrasting vividly with the patients' social personality and way of life. They often experience it as ego-dystonic, alien, embarrassing, not belonging to them and split off. Early, pre-oedipal anxieties do not predominate here; the basic problem is essentially a susceptible and vulnerable masculinity. This is where the "motivational priority" in Stolorow's sense (cf 1979, p. 41) comes in. One form of expression of this masculinity problem is inhibition, denial of phallic aggression which is exclusively or mainly bound into the symptom and so acquires the function of protecting objects and sustaining an ordered way of life. The key problem here seems to be contraphobic coping with castration anxiety originating from the unresolved oedipal conflict, which earlier psychoanalytical literature placed too closely at the centre of perversion theory and which more recent perversion literature, by contrast, often simply ignores as something marginal or superficial.

In one respect these patients are well-equipped for *psychotherapy*, being so-cially stable, having a circumscribed symptom, no severe structural disorders and above all being capable of entering into relationships. On the other hand therapeutic contact can be impeded if these patients experience their symptom which contrasts so strikingly with their self-image, as something extremely alien to their ego and show little awareness of this contradiction. The result can be considerable resistance to questioning their own one-sided image of themselves as this entails giving up the tendency to deny the existence of any conflicts.

This group is represented in Cases 2 and 14 and is exemplified in the follow-ing case history.

Case 15

The 25-year-old patient had been charged with exposing himself to young women. He fough for an opportunity to get therapy with great vigour and perseverance, as he was worried by the pending trial.

He is a casually dressed, seemingly boyish and intelligent young man of medium height; he is well-mannered and polite.

He comes from a middle-class family. His father, editor of a small newspaper, was only interested in his profession and had little time for his family so that the mother turned all he loving attention onto the son. He describes her as being a lively woman who was sociable and attractive. She took great care of him and paved the way for him. He was his mother's pride and pet. He never got into difficulties with his parents because he always complied, in contras to his elder sister who left home early after quarrelling with them. Family life was marked by a tendency to avoid conflict, much emphasis on being friendly and a complete taboo on sexuality. After leaving secondary school he trained for a commercial job where he was respected and worked his way up to become branch manager. He has many acquaintances, teache sports as a sideline and is liked by everybody.

Prior to marriage he initially had potency problems in relationships with girls; he though he was a failure and so avoided sexual contacts. He has been married for 3 years; he describe his marriage as being happy. Sexual dysfunctions only occur rarely. His wife is in charge and does everything for him, just like his mother. His fairness and boyishness are greatly appreciated in all his activities and interest areas, particularly on the sports field. He avoids competing with others and even tends to back down, a technique he uses with great success. Thi gives him the self-confidence he lacks in sexual matters where he feels vulnerable and uncertain of himself.

Since puberty he has felt the urge to expose himself occasionally. He suffers from this and sees it as something alien, like an illness which has nothing to do with him.

Psychodynamic Aspects: The patient has succeeded in becoming self-reliant, despite being th apple of his mother's eye, and in living a successful professional and social life. His problem can be narrowed down to the vulnerability of his male identity. His psychosexual development is anchored in the oedipal love for his mother with the concomitant phantasy of not being sexually adequate. He is uncertain about his sexual potency and cannot assert himself in manly fashion. The *symptom* is an attempt to cope contraphobically with his castration anxiet by demonstrating and convincing himself of his phallic potency and intactness.

Therapy see p. 93.

3.6.2 Depressive Patients (Cluster 2)

The patients in this group, like those in clusters 3 and 4, rate as moderately disturbed in the *description of variables* (see Table 7). A markedly negative self-image, a depressive view on life, occasional potency disorders and thoughts of committing suicide are characteristic of this group. Symptoms such as psychosomatic complaints and alcoholism were seen in only some patients. There is no consistent pattern of aggression problems. Social integration is not as smooth and harmonious as in the first group; the patients are more labile, socially more on the fringe but not outsiders; there is almost no criminality. The deviancy has taken firm hold, is in some cases increasingly insistent and generally more pronounced than in the first group; no violent sexual offences have been committed.

In contrast to cluster 1, the main characteristic of patients in this group is not a definable oedipal problem. The most noticeable aspect is the difficulty they have in maintaining their self-esteem. A negative self-image with pervasive feelings of being good for nothing, ineffectual, inadequate, which can verge on the suicidal, is typical. Compared with cluster 1, the development of their autonomy has been obstructed more severely. While patients in the first group developed a male identity, even though it proved vulnerable, in these patients the foundations of male identity are more frail; potency disorders are pathognomic. Their anxieties about their masculinity have less to do with castration fears than with body image problems. Their aggression is directed largely against themselves. Their depressive attitudes signal that they feel helpless and destitute, that they find themselves hard to bear. They tend to succumb to dependency and let themselves be looked after by others (significant correlation with coping strategies seeking dependency; $p < 1\%$). They seek support, comfort, a boost to their shaky self-esteem and, in relationships, tend toward childlike dependency. Separation anxieties and fear of abandonment are of key significance.

Their *symptom,* which is in some a "perverse reaction" and in others the expression of a fixed perversion, plays a more important role and is more pressing than in group 1. They are mainly exhibitionists and nonviolent pedophiles, and their acting out tends to be more regressive than aggressive. The perverse symptom is linked less to a feeling of power and potency than to a need for consolation, to fill up an inner void, the sexualized gratification of pre-oedipal oral needs. The perverse symptom counterbalances their depressive tendencies and enables them to experience themselves very intensely for a moment; at the same time, however, it reinforces their negative opinion of themselves as it is a highly ego-dystonic and conflict-ridden form of coping. The patient feels guilty and ashamed and regards his symptom as a confirmation of his utter worthlessness.

In *psychotherapy* this group proved the most accessible of all the patients. This was because they sought help, needed support, were at odds with themselves independently of the symptom and were therefore openly prepared to enter into a therapeutic process. As their coping strategies and defence mechanisms were not as successful as in the first patient group, they also showed less resistance to questioning their own motives. The problem for the therapist was to avoid being distracted by the patient's deep desire to become dependent on and idealize him.

Case 16

The 38-year-old patient came to therapy on a court order and had been repeatedly convicted for indecent exposure to children.

He is small, corpulent, very stylishly dressed and makes a reticent impression. One senses his deep apprehension about revealing himself and his fear of being rebuffed or even despised.

His childhood was unsettled. During the war his family had to flee from home. He lost his father at an early age and his mother married again, but lost her second husband a few years later. It was very difficult to make ends meet. The family tried settling in the GDR but as they were refugees they were socially ostracized. He describes his mother as being a difficult woman who was moody and unpredictable. She would treat him affectionately, but then suddenly became hard and strict with him - something he could not understand. As he grew older he felt restricted, watched-over and exploited by her. He more or less fled from her to West Germany. After his poverty-stricken childhood he dreamt of earning enough money to live an independent, free life. He moved from place to place, was rootless and initially had difficulty finding work.

He has an uneasy attitude towards his body: he feels ugly and is extremely bashful. He had sexual experiences with girls at a relatively early age, but they proved to be short-lived and noncommittal. He frequently has erection problems. He has only once had a steady girlfriend who soon left him. He was very jealous, tried to dominate, restrict and control his girlfriend and make her dependent on him. When she put up resistance he became aggressive towards her. After the separation he was deeply depressed and has never got involved in a close relationship since. He is afraid both of being abandoned and of being dominated by women, and also of his own aggression which could evolve out of his disappointment. Over the last 12 years he has had no relationship at all and has been living alone as a permanent guest in a small hotel. He feels lonely and depressive, useless and unloved. Professionally he is a success: he works a great deal and is proud of his achievements. However, he is very sensitive in dealings with colleagues and easily loses his temper when he feels insulted. As a consequence people avoid him. As he cannot stand being alone he very often goes to bars, drinks a lot and is in danger of becoming an alcoholic.

After the separation from his girlfriend he began exposing himself to small girls. He condemns his behaviour, feels he is a "lousy rat" and is very ashamed. He has difficulty talking about this problem.

Psychodynamic Aspects: This patient's development is marked by fundamental insecurity: anxiety, the loss of two fathers, refugee life, his emotionally unreliable mother - all this gave him little inner stability. His self-esteem and male identity are vulnerable. His relationships failed because of his wish for complete protection and exclusiveness; after that he went into "voluntary solitary exile" to protect himself from further disappointments. His professional success guarantees him a certain self-assurance, but his craving to be loved remains unappeased. The *symptom* emerged after he had been deserted, his hope of intimacy and protection had been crushed, and he felt insulted, rebuffed and debased as a man. Showing his penis to a child audience enables him to restore his damaged masculinity and compensate for his loneliness and inner emptiness. While feeling he is not a match for women, he can experience his potency with children without running the risk of being despised.

Therapy see p. 125.

3.6.3 Patients with Marked Defences Against Depression (Cluster 3)

In terms of the *description of variables* (see Table 7) the patients in this group were assessed as moderately disturbed, as in cluster 2. Their ability to relate to others is more restricted, as a rule their view on life is not, or only slightly, depressive. Their aggression potential is high, control of aggression low; nevertheless, aggression hardly plays any role in their offences. Some are socially well integrated, others less so. They show a significant preference for coping strategies in which they repeatedly enter into new relationships ($p < 1\%$). As with cluster 2, the deviancy is firmly established but shows no signs of becoming more severe. Symptoms such as alcoholism, psychosomatic disorders and criminality are characteristic for this group and are always present, frequently in combination.

Whereas it is characteristic of cluster 2 to show a depressive need for support and dependency, in this group unstable relationships, defence against depression, somatic symptoms and criminal acting out are typical. The perversion itself also seems to defend the patient from falling into a depression. Put rather crudely, this group represents the opposite face of the "depressive" type, the essential differences lying in their emotional resilience, coping with aggression and relating to others. They do not look on the dark side of life; sorrow, despair and anxieties are not evident; all of them use alcohol to alleviate emotional tension.

The patients' basic problem is an inability to feel depressed, and they often convey a superficial impression of strong-mindedness and autonomy. They defend themselves by launching a counterattack; they see themselves in single combat, and demonstrate a strength of purpose which covers up their fears and vulnerability. Avoiding commitment in relationships is a kind of protective shield: intimacy soon makes them feel naked and at the mercy of the other person. It is typical of them to avoid introspection and deny they have any problems. Inner tensions are acted out extrapsychically in the form of antisocial outbursts and/or as psychosomatic symptoms. They also avoid dealing with the conflicts underlying the perverse symptom. Whereas the patients in group 2 deal with their conflicts autoplastically and neurotically, this group tends to externalize and act out in order to restore their intrapsychic homeoostasis, reinstate their damaged self-esteem or compensate losses.

The initial blatant discrepancy between their relatively good social integration and their criminality is explained by a remarkable phenomenon we observed in a number of patients: in their youth their behaviour is predominantly antisocial and criminal; once they have overcome this criminality, frequently with the help of a stabilizing environment, the perverse symptom emerges, gains importance or persists. Our interpretation of such *changes in the symptom* is that aggressive tensions are no longer acted out alloplastically, but are sexualized, contained and defused in the perverse symptom; at the same time the patient becomes more skilled in adapting socially. We observed this phenomenon in Case 13 and in the following case history, which is typical for group 3.

Case 17

The 34-year-old patient was sent to us by the court for treatment after being discovered exposing himself to women several times.

He is a broad-shouldered, muscular man who at first sight radiates calm, humour and a genial manner

His father, a sailor, divorced his mother when he was still a small child. He lived with his grandparents for a while, felt happy there and had a good relationship with his grandfather. He describes the latter as being a calm, warm-hearted person who was not easily ruffled or upset by his moody, cantankerous wife. He met his father for the first time at age 14 and went to live with him because his elderly grandparents could not take care of him any longer. He could not get on with his father who he describes as being short-tempered and strict. He rebelled against him, committed small thefts and was temporarily put in a home. Authority problems continued: he always had difficulties with his superiors, refused to accept what others told him, was quick to feel patronized - a situation he resisted defiantly. After the home he went back to his mother. He developed a very close relationship to her; she was always loyal to him, helped him find his bearings and gain a foothold in life.

As a child he was timorous, shy and frail. He suffered for a time from bronchial asthma. At school he was afraid of being laughed at when trying to make friends. He overcame his shyness by acting as the class clown, but inwardly he still felt alone. He read countless adventure and detective stories and identified with the heroes. After secondary school he broke off an apprenticeship after a dispute with his boss. He worked in the docks, got into criminal circles and committed a series of burglaries. Testing his courage and looking for adventure were important factors. He was repeatedly convicted and spent a total of 7 years in jail. In recent years he has moved away from this milieu. In the docks he worked his way up to a senior position. Hard physical work is important for him; he needs the feeling of getting to grips with and succeeding in a task. Now that he no longer has superiors he gets on well at work.

Since puberty he has had a pronounced preference for older, maternal women. The relationships never last long as he soon feels cramped and restricted. He avoids closer contact to other people, just socializing with colleagues, neighbours or acquaintances. He only opens up after drinking large quantities of alcohol. For the last 3 years he has been married to an older woman who has three daughters. His role as father and provider fills him with pride; he gives and finds support in home life. He has little in common with his wife. Conflicts and arguments do not occur as he is afraid of losing this laboriously acquired stability after so many years of rootlessness.

His exhibitionist problem has existed since puberty. He is intensely ashamed, as this kind of behaviour is irreconcilable with his male ideal of strength, superiority and independence. His need to expose himself is occasionally compulsive and often connected with heavy drinking. In recent years he has exposed himself particularly at times of hidden tension between him and his wife when he felt inwardly angry and dissatisfied. He wants to "get rid" of his symptom and sees it as "the only weakness I cannot cope with".

Pschodynamic Aspects: This patient seeks refuge from his deep, hidden doubts about his own masculinity by fighting a head-on battle with them: he subjects himself to tests of courage which threaten his social existence; he joins a social milieu in which showing weakness is forbidden and reacts touchily and aggressively to anything that appears to undermine his strength. Despite setbacks he always manages to assert himself, often investing considerable physical effort. This stereotype, "strongman" behaviour conceals a deep desire for maternal care which, however, soon seems to be a threat as it undermines his own independence. With the *symptom* he has to reassure himself of his masculinity and potency; it is a protest against the insulting role of a small boy who needs a mother to give his life stability and a proper hold. It expresses the complete collapse of an energetic attempt to assert himself, a fight against the feeling of being weak and defenceless.

Therapy, see p. 91.

3.6.4 Noninterpretable Group (Cluster 4)

The profile of this group seems less clear and cannot really be interpreted (see Table 7). This result is important as it demonstrates that the 4 interpretable clusters by no means cover the entire spectrum of heterogeneity - especially as this cluster contains 12 patients.

3.6.5 Severely Disturbed Social Outsiders (Cluster 5)

In our *description of variables* (cf. Table 7) patients in this group are assessed as severely pathological. They are mostly incapable of relating to others; various types of disorder mar their perception of themselves; many harbour grandiose phantasies. Their lives are chaotic and unstructured: lack of social ties, considerable potential for aggression, poor aggression control, alcoholism, psychosomatic disturbances, suicidal tendencies, potency disorders and criminality are factors in almost all these patients. The deviancy has become more severe; offences are almost always violent and linked with omnipotence phantasies ($C = 0.48$). This group consists almost entirely of patients who committed aggressive pedophile offences and sexually aggressive acts against women. Most of the patients showed symptoms of deprivation, antisocial and psychopathic behaviour, superego defects and severe personality disturbances verging on a borderline pathology. Coping strategies involving direct or indirect use of aggression and of avoiding dependency were significantly more frequent.

The offences committed by these patients always involve a discharge of sexualized aggression. In cluster 5 *aggressive sexual perversions* and *aggressive impulse neuroses* are combined; the psychodynamics of these phenomena have been described by Schorsch and Becker (1977). Both have common psychodynamic roots in early disturbances in the development of drives, ego and self. Deep-seated anxieties of annihilation, destruction and an inner void interact with considerable aggressively charged narcissistic tension. The defence mechanism *perversion formation* works by sexualizing unneutralized destructive impulses and narcissistic configurations (illusions of grandeur) and binding them into the perversion, so that they are sucked up by it. This relief is missing in *impulsive acts*. These patients are typically fixed in the "schizoid position" in Klein's (1932) sense (see Sect. 3.2.2) in which fears of being destroyed are overcome by means of archaic splitting processes while reality is perceived in a radically distorted manner. The patients' almost paranoid reactions show how important projective mechanisms are. Attempts at relationships fail already in the early phases because fragments of the early mother-child relationship are projectively brought to life in the partner; this induces in part a yearning for fusion with the good mother imago, in part a hate-ridden acting out against the evil imagines. Narcissistic tension and unease induced by a constant dread of losing identity are permanently present and have to be answered by illusions of grandeur and omnipotence which act either permanently or temporarily (in crises) as a way of coping with feelings of defencelessness, helplessness and total emptiness.

Of course, these patients present the most problems *in therapy.* We shall, however, demonstrate that constructive therapy is, within limits, possible.

Case 18

This 20-year-old patient was referred to us from a state psychiatric hospital. He had been sentenced to 2½ years confinement for several aggressive sexual attacks on prepubertal girls, some involving extreme violence.

The patient seems younger than he is and at first presents himself as harmless, childish, confiding and in need of help. Gradually it becomes obvious that he is at heart deeply suspicious, uses his helplessness extortionately and is emotionally far further out of reach and less easily approachable than at first seems the case.

He grew up in a chaotic environment: his family lives on the fringe of society, his father was an alcoholic, uncontrolled, hot-tempered, aggressive and had been convicted for several offences. He assumed the role of a guest in the family; when he was at home everyone was afraid of him. The family also housed a grandmother, mother and 5 other siblings who also showed symptoms of deprivation. Two brothers had been convicted for rape. The atmosphere in the family was highly charged and tense. New alliances, involving the children as well, were constantly formed within the family. In the first years of his life the patient was mainly looked after by his grandmother who spoilt him materially. His mother then drew him onto her side, pampered him and was at the same time seductive, slept in the same bed with him and used him as a kind of weapon in her fights with his father. Behavioural disorders such as enuresis and encopresis developed. At the age of 9 his parent's house burned down. He dramatizes the story by misleadingly claiming that three of his brothers and sisters and the entire animal stock died in the fire. Symptoms of neglect emerged early on in the form of thefts and playing truant. When the youth welfare office intervened, his mother shielded him and threatened to kill both herself and her son if they took him away from her. He was nonetheless confined to a home. His mother, suspecting the father was behind it all, encouraged him to rebel against the home. The patient was unable to fit in. Initially, it was said he had great difficulty relating to others and was very nervous; later he was described as a troublemaker, an aggressive rowdy who beat up his juniors. Criminal charges brought against him at about the age of 14 for a number of thefts and also for sexually aggressive acts against small girls, whom he had choked and raped, were dropped as he had not reached the age of discretion. As the home was unable to cope with him any longer, he was given back to his mother. His apprenticeship was interrupted by new sex offences. He was deemed unfit to plead (Section 20, German penal code) and committed to a state psychiatric hospital. During his apprenticeship he had a girlfriend for a short while, but he found sex with her less stimulating than his contacts with small girls. He had homosexual experiences both at the home and in hospital, but prefers not to talk about them.

Psychodynamic Aspects: This is a patient who grew up without any long-term guiding authority and possesses practically no strategies enabling him to cope with real life. In the family drama, in desolate conditions on the outskirts of society, he was used by his mother in her battle against the hated father for her own ends and then dropped again. The complete lack of any sympathetic understanding in the past is reflected in his inability to empathize or adjust to others. He functionalizes his environment in his own interests and demands to be taken care of as he was never granted the right to be self-reliant. He is deeply suspicious and feels constantly threatened, which induces him to redraw reality pseudologistically so he can feel more important and influential. Aggressively destructive and sexual impulses are fused and used as a defence against being powerless and on the verge of being destroyed. The *symptom* does not function as a circumscribed conflict-solving strategy, but is part of an aimless, chaotic acting out, a vehicle for his destructive impulses and his hatred, among other things. It gives him a feeling of potency and power and the opportunity to dispose projectively of the deep-rooted notion of his own childishness and weakness.

Therapy, see p. 126.

4 Therapy

4.1 Formal Framework

In describing the formal framework of therapy we are faced with a problem typical of practice-oriented psychotherapy research: growing experience increases one's doubts in the original concept and makes modifications necessary (see Sect. 1.2). To convey the full scope of the experience we made, we shall also mention some therapeutic procedures which proved not to be particularly helpful.

Therapy was conducted between 1974 and 1981 by four female and five male psychologists with training in behaviour therapy and client-centred psychotherapy. Continuous supervision was provided by a Balint group and regular team discussions. The *therapy team* always consisted of four to five psychologists of whom half were employed full-time on the project and half on a fee basis. The relatively high fluctuation of therapists was not only due to therapists' changing jobs, but also to the fact that working exclusively or mainly with these patients put a great strain on the therapists.

Our initial concern with the degree of influence exerted by *the sex of the therapist* on therapy was gradually relativized in the course of our work. Generally speaking, psychotherapy for sex offenders does not differ much from psychotherapy for other patients. The decision in favour of a male or female therapist is no more of a problem than with other patients and, assuming one has enough personnel to even discuss alternatives, can be based on analogous criteria. However, we have not ignored the fact that, as in other therapies, the therapist's sex gives the therapeutic relationship and developing dynamics a specific character. Although we gave thought to the influence of the therapist's sex when assigning patients to male or female therapists, we were not able to analyse the effects systematically owing to lack of personnel. Patients were assigned to therapists depending on their availability and independently of sex. Retrospective analysis showed that distribution was random: there were no significant correlations between the patients' characteristics prior to therapy and the sex of the therapist, nor beween the therapist's sex and the outcome of therapy. Patients who wanted to enact a perverse symptom in front of a female therapist were the exception (two exhibitionists). We soon discovered that this was a provocative acting out in critical phases of therapy.

Duration of therapy was generally between 1 and 2 years with 35 to 60 therapy hours and one session per week.

At the start of the project, when the focus was more on behaviour therapy methods, we treated out-of-town patients on an inpatient basis over 4 to 8 weeks. However, under these conditions we found it difficult to approach problems effectively, especially as we had no ward of our own and planned treatment on an outpatient basis could not be continued. We therefore consider this setting unsatisfactory.

About two thirds of the therapies were *individual therapy*. In many cases the patient's partner was asked to join therapy although this could not be termed continuous couple therapy. Individual and couple therapy were combined in one fifth of the therapies. As a rule a therapist of the opposite sex was added to a *couple therapy* group. Patients seldom underwent only couple therapy.

Positive reports in the literature (see, for example, Mathis and Collins 1970, and Giese and Kober 1983) encouraged us to conduct three *group therapies* - partly as the only therapy, partly in combination with individual therapy. Efforts focussed on social learning in the sense of assertion training. We were not able to motivate patients to take part regularly or to initiate a constructive group process. We asked ourselves why we were unable to replicate the positive results achieved elsewhere and believe that this was probably due to our patient sample. Group therapy was indicated for patients with poor social skills; however, we did not always appreciate how frequently their poor social integration stemmed from serious problems in relating to others, which explained their initially low motivation for group therapy. In fact, these patients tended to hide in the group. In this case the common problems separated the patients instead of joining them.

Although Petri (1980) reported positively on combining anti-androgens and psychotherapy, we dispensed with suppression of sexual drive through anti-androgen medication. The exceptions were six patients whose probation prescribed *anti-androgen treatment*. Even so we soon stopped medication; in the shelter of therapy this proved to make sense and was usually accepted by the courts. The reason for dispensing with such treatment was that we had observed that it can by itself have serious and not easily calculable "psychotherapeutic" effects. It can assume the function of an introjected prosthesis or crutch and encourage the patient to experience his drives as independent egodystonic forces or fixate the patient on this kind of problem handling; as a result the key problem becomes inaccessible to therapy. Anti-androgen medication can also activate the patient's tendency to inflict punishment on himself and reinforce castration anxieties (see also Sigusch 1980). For our patients, at least, these considerations seemed to us more important as a starting point for therapy than the relief from "sexual drive" and the acute danger of relapse which Petri emphasized. We were impressed to see how patients, who initially experienced their instinctual impulses as being almost uncontrollably compulsive and quasi automatic, changed their perception during therapy - when, that is, a stable patient-therapist relationship had developed.

Following therapy (3.9 years had elapsed on average by the closing date, April 1982) one fifth of the patients were given intensive aftercare sessions particularly in relapse cases or to prevent relapse. With these patients, more s than with others, it is imperative to offer further therapeutic support, even afte therapy and after they have more or less stabilized. This opportunity was use more often by these patients than we had expected from our experience wit other patient groups. One factor may have been that patients experienced th trust and continuity in therapy as an emotional corrective to their earlier sepa ration and abandonment traumata, but were at first unable to apply this experi ence elsewhere. This is why patients continually have to reassure themselves o this possibility, especially in crises. It is important for the patients to have permanent "port of call" where they can expect help when they need it. Ou patients were usually quite willing to continue therapy with a new discussio partner when the previous therapist was no longer available.

Case 2 (see p. 34 for history)

The patient was treated in four phases, each lasting 1–2 years with intervals of several month During the first 2 years the patient was treated by a woman. Although he managed to unde stand his strategies and control symptoms, the patient was unable to lower his defences wit the therapist: reinforced by the behaviour therapy arrangement, the traumatizing pattern of h relationship to a dominating, strict mother constantly recurred. This became evident whe therapy was continued in the second phase with a male therapist to whom he soon develope a trusting relationship. Treatment proceeded in a distinctly more relaxed atmosphere. Onl then did the symptom's context become clearer. The patient cooperated by, for instance, n longer drinking alcohol. For the first time the patient was able to talk to the therapist openl about his sexual inhibitions, his masturbation scruples, his feeling of having a damaged bod At the end of this phase the patient believed he had overcome his exhibitionist desires whic now played only a subordinate role in his phantasies.

After the birth of his first child (a son) he relapsed again. He was proud of his role as fathe but was afraid he could not measure up to it. The notion that his son might, like himself, als become an exhibitionist filled him with panic. After a few crisis sessions he stabilized again. relapse occurred a year later and sessions were resumed; the patient had been promoted work and was afraid he would be unable to meet the increasing demands. It again became ev dent how much the patient needed his symptom as a crutch for his vulnerable masculinity.

At follow-up 2 years after the last therapy session the patient reported occasional exhib tionist desires in crises which he did not, however, have to enact. He was satisfied and made confident and composed impression on the therapist.

In summary, for the patient treatment meant primarily support and stabilization of a ma identity highly susceptible to crises, especially in the phases with the male therapist. Apa from learning methods of self-control, it was important that he understood his symptom; relapses he was able to work through his compulsive need to repeat this act of "self-sabotage It was important for the patient to experience the therapist as an understanding father/broth who encouraged him and as someone he could accept.

4.2 Motivation for Therapy: A Discussion

There is broad consensus in psychotherapy research that patient self-motiv tion, with the two dimensions distress and acceptance of the illness, is a sir qua non of successful psychotherapy. In practical terms this means, for exan ple, that obstacles inherent in the health service (such as long waiting time high costs, etc.) are in a way positively interpreted and count as a test of the patient's motivation and, consequently, as positive selection criteria. This may be valid for the classical psychotherapeutic setting as the initial problems are clear: a patient has conflicts, inhibitions, anxieties, impairments to his wellbeing, etc. - i. e. symptoms mostly experienced *intrapsychically*. Only when the patient actually suffers and the patient shows signs of being willing to work with the therapist is psychotherapy indicated.

This is no longer true once psychotherapy is attempted with fringe groups, especially when symptoms or conflicts are experienced less intrapsychically, but are instead *acted out extrapsychically* and this acting out also takes the form of anti- or asocial behaviour. Generally, one of the dimensions of motivation (*acceptance of illness*) is missing in a double sense: both the patients themselves and their environment judge deviant sexual behaviour primarily by moral standards. Moreover, it is often doubted or questioned whether they experience the other dimension distress. It is doubtful whether psychotherapists really are free of prejudice and values when assessing patients; the fact that there are hardly any systematic studies on this topic in the relevant literature speaks for itself.

Sexual delinquents seeking help from a therapist, usually under pressure of actual or feared sanctions, are often rejected with the argument that psychotherapy is only feasible on a strictly voluntary basis without external pressure. Further, as perverse acts imply feelings of pleasure delinquents can at most suffer from the social consequences and not from the acts themselves. If one insists on expecting patients to motivate themselves in advance, moral aspects are involved: some kind of confession of guilt or moral self-condemnation is expected (see Appelbaum 1972). This can block the therapist's access to the patient and the patient's access to therapy.

The reasons for the need to revise this concept of motivation can firstly be found in the *objective circumstances prior to therapy* which are scarcely comparable to those in classical psychotherapy, either for patients or for therapists. Second, there are *specific difficulties in initiating a relationship between therapist and patient* which cannot be traced to the patient's problems alone but are equally rooted in the situation the patient and therapist find themselves in.

4.2.1 Special Circumstances Prior to Therapy

When discussing the motivation problem it is important to recognize that considerable difficulties for both patients and therapists arise prior to therapy.

Before therapy the *patient's* difficulties consist essentially of being understood with his affliction; the symptom provokes rejection and outrage and does more to conceal his problem than to show it. To understand the problem of motivation it is important to find out not only what function the symptom has in the patient's life, which deficits it makes up for, but also which factors obstruct therapy. We described how in the perverse ritual patients triumph over and recompensate for previous traumata and may experience great elation coupled with momentary physical pleasure. However, it would be short-sighted t take this as an argument for a lack of distress. Assessing the symptom out c context, as a kind of thing unto itself is highly artificial and antitherapeutic. I one examines the patient's general problems in which the symptom is beddec one is often confronted with profound misery, loneliness and isolation, self-de nial, loss of self-esteem and the pain of a loveless sexuality which frequentl forces the patient to lead a tormenting double existence or pushes him onto th very edge of society.

One of the many paradoxes of an ideology which takes a permissive attitud towards sexuality is that it discriminates against people whose deviant sexu behaviour has become manifest. This blinds one to the fact that they usuall have an extremely inhibited and anxious attitude towards sexuality and are o ten ashamed of, frightened and puzzled by their sexual impulses which brea all the social rules. These people are under double pressure from both their fe of public sanctions and the loss of control over themselves which induces pe plexity, anxieties, guilt feelings, depression and even suicide attempts. In ou opinion, it is bordering on cynicism to question the suffering of a man who i afraid of being prosecuted and of his perversion being discovered, as th would involve not only loss of social prestige, but also the loss of his sel respect. It is a grave narcissistic insult for anyone to find out that he is not h own master, to be aware of something in him which can neither be reconcile with his self-image nor controlled. For reasons they cannot understand, but o ly vaguely sense, many of these patients live with a more or less extreme an tormenting dependence on their symptom. Particularly as regards self-respec we consider it important to find out why patients with deviant sexuality rel tively seldom ask for help spontaneously. Most of them live with their perve sion in secret and conceal it even from their most intimate partners, if they a not already completely isolated. How difficult it must be to take one's sym toms to an anonymous institution where one cannot be sure whether one's ow degradation might not be intensified still further by sheer lack of understandin or perhaps even punishment! The biographies of many patients tell of appal ing experiences with authorities and experts; they are consequently afraid new confrontations. Furthermore, very few know about the rare opportuniti available for pychotherapeutic help with sexual problems.

The *therapist's* motivation is also influenced by the objective circumstanc prior to therapy. Therapists working with patients whose symptoms ha caused them to come in conflict with the law find themselves in a situatio which presents a difficult challenge to their therapeutic identity. Any thera with criminals starts off in a *paradox situation*; the general setting is *antither peutic.* Those in charge of enforcing the law and other institutions of public a thority are watching in the background. They keep a careful eye not only on t patient in his social context, but also on the therapist in his work, which has be successful. This is evident in every phase: the court enquires whether ther py is progressing, the police reports new offences, lawyers and courts want e pert evidence, probation officers intervene or are called upon for advice.

Under these circumstances it is particularly difficult for a therapist to find her/his bearings and maintain her/his *therapeutic identity*. In this context, maintaining therapeutic identity means viewing the symptom not as a punishable offence, but understanding its psychodynamic function and so finding access to the underlying problems and the patient's need for help. Being at the centre of attention of criminal offender, social norms, law enforcement and victims, the therapist's highest priority must be *loyalty to the patient*. This loyalty should not be mistaken for blind complicity in which patient and therapist could jointly ignore social norms or the victim's situation. Consequently, it involves potential conflict for the therapist. This loyality is all the more difficult to sustain the more violent the offence is, the more damaging its assessed effect on the victim and (aside from potential harm to others) the more the therapist's fears are mobilized by any conflict with his/her own norms and values.

One can see that not only the patient, but also the therapist encounters circumstances prior to treatment which are liable to undermine the motivation of both. This may well be the reason why many therapists doubt the patient's motivation for therapy and consequently projectively free themselves of the burden of treatment. If the patient is willing, however, the situation described presents special dangers which can distort the therapeutic situation from the start. This can happen, for instance, if the therapist reacts with exaggerated eagerness and feels compelled to assume the initiative and responsibility, to get involved and to have an effect. Since his image of himself as a therapist includes the conviction that therapy is a meaningful alternative to senseless imprisonment, he/she has to prove that it really is effective.

4.2.2 The First Encounter Between Patient and Therapist

We can summarize the *general contradiction in circumstances prior to therapy* as follows: both the therapist and the patient are at least superficially in the same situation; they meet at the instigation of others with the task of dealing with the patient's socially undesirable behaviour. Both are dependent and under surveillance; the therapist is saddled with the responsibility by both sides: by society's legal institutions and by the patient. The situation is initially antitherapeutic.

The *first contact* between patient and therapist is naturally also influenced by this situation. This means that the therapist has to concede the patient his *mistrust*; in the patient's eyes the therapist is after all the representative or at least the agent of the institutions condemning or persecuting him. This situation alone confronts the therapist with a difficult problem. Every therapist, and particularly the less experienced, will experience a meeting with a patient whose attitude is at first sceptical as a rebuffal and insult. This can provoke reactions which may impede or even thwart the therapeutic process.

- The patient's mistrust may be blamed on his lack of motivation.
- The danger is, moreover, that the therapist will team up with the patier against the institutions, their mutual "evil persecutor". The therapist is all th more likely to do so if he feels the state authorities are repressive and an ot stacle to his work. This alliance involves self-deception and relinquishing im portant therapeutic advantages: the therapist actually provokes the patier into manipulating him and forcing decisions out of him. At the same time h misses the opportunity to act as a guiding example for the patient.
- Another ineffective means of reducing the patient's mistrust, apart fror emotional reserve and complicity, is to play down or deny the fact that bot really are dependent on outside forces.
- In his confusion the therapist may also attempt to ignore the patient's scept cism or disapproval by acting out social control in the guise of therapy and for example, devote himself to rigorous removal of the symptom using equa ly strict techniques.

It is not only the objective circumstances - which cannot be compared to thos in normal psychotherapy - which entice therapist and patient to enter into fruitless collusion. Because of their *problems* the patients often behave in way which affect therapy motivation and can only be understood in psychodynami terms; these too help to shape the initial contact. Although the heterogeneity c the patients precludes any reference to "the" sex offender as such, we shall de scribe a few *characteristic features* for clarity's sake.

Some of our patients were comparable with traditional psychotherapy pa tients in terms of social background, education and introspective ability. The were also deeply distressed and were highly motivated for therapy. Workin with them was rewarding; nevertheless, they represent a minority.

Difficulties arise in therapy for patients from *lower social classes* with les well-developed introspective abilities. About two thirds of our patients had n idea what psychotherapy meant. They associated therapy with somatic inte vention, with something they passively let happen to them.

This attitude can only partly be explained by their social background; th main cause lies in the patients' central dilemma. "Criminal acting out" of inne conflicts always contains an element of acting out attacks against and oppos tion to powerful authorities. Infringing on taboos and norms is a kind of provo cation and implies that a counterreaction in the form of anger, persecution c punishment of some kind is expected. These reactions are, so to speak, a calcu lated risk in the perverse act. This is what Stoller (1975) means when he re marks that the desire to face risk and danger is a specific quality of pervers pleasure. Seen in this light, the remarkably weak resistance these patients sho to drastic "offers of treatment" such as castration, brain surgery and suppres sion of sex drive is quite intelligible; such treatment fits in with their patholog

This factor is also always present in the initial meeting with the therapist an can take different forms: the patient may, for example, start to fear, expect an need punishment, or he may try repeatedly escaping from the "persecutors and the therapist to gain a feeling of grandiose superiority.

All these factors result in the patient taking a *passively receptive attitude* to a therapeutic situation which is unfamiliar and consequently open to the widest variety of phantasies. Perceiving the therapist initially as an authority and a potential source of punishment triggers not only negative reactions such as suspicion, reserve and a tendency to hide, but also positive hopes in the patient.

A passive, receptive attitude of this kind can even lead to *hope of a magic cure* by imagining the powerful therapist is in a position to conjure away the symptom. This attitude is boosted by ego-dystonic coping when the symptom is experienced as alien to the ego, as something which does not belong to the self or is regarded as highly unwelcome. This childlike, magical exaggeration can present the therapist with dangers as well as opportunities. He may, for example, feel encouraged to live up to the patient's expectations. In doing so he becomes dependent and reacts to the inevitable disappointment with feelings of guilt and insufficiency, which then distort his relationship to the patient. Alternatively, he can unthinkingly exert his power over the patient which can lead to dependency or failure to reach him. His chance is to pick up the patient's positive offer of a relationship in which the unrealistic aspects can be discussed and dealt with.

If fears of punishment prevail, the patient articulates this magical thinking not, or not so much, as hope of a magic cure, but more as *fear of being subtly manipulated* - which one patient termed "fear of being brainwashed".

The idea that therapy is something which happens to you as a patient can be acted out not just by passively waiting for it, but also by actively resisting it. If the therapeutic relationship is pervaded by this *resistant acting out* a pseudotherapy evolves. These patients manipulate the therapist by pretending to cooperate so as to "earn" the social benefits they hope to claim with medical certificates, recommendations etc. The therapist, who can all too easily become the victim of his own pity, soon feels misused and functionalized, i.e. reduced to a function. However, it is important to realize that this functionalizing is frequently an element in initial contacts and can express an understandable and *legitimate claim*. The therapist is not only, and often not primarily, expected to provide help in dealing with intrapsychic problems but also, and sometimes mainly, an authority who can cope with practical problems: protection from or alternatives to being confined in a psychiatric hospital; help in finding an apartment, a job, requalifying for a driving licence, etc.; these are often critical and existentially important concerns for the patient. Even though solving these existential problems should not be the only concern of therapy and the therapist should not take on these social tasks himself, but rather delegate them if possible to a social worker, he should be prepared to offer support in the form of certificates, reports and the like. Therapists who already feel they are being used when they do this and who barricade themselves behind therapeutic abstinence or restrict themselves to verbalizing the emotional aspects these problems involve, block their own and the patient's path to therapy.

Another major problem in the initial encounter is *making the symptom a topic for discussion* - something the patient may expect and be afraid of, for several reasons:

Strong *feelings of shame and guilt* connected with the symptom can imped the establishment of a therapeutic relationship. If the patient manages to gai some trust in the therapist and can communicate the distressing feelings linke to the symptom in the first sessions, the emotional relief he feels can become a important driving force in therapy. Some patients are incapable of overcomin their enormous embarrassment at talking about a symptom which further re duces their already low self-esteem and can only do so after a minimum of trus in the therapist has developed. Unless the therapist handles the patient wit caution and respects this sensitive barrier, he runs the risk of failing. The pa tient will then either stay away or, if he still comes, will be taciturn and with drawn and the therapeutic relationship will remain hollow. Despite the incisiv and painful consequences, other patients feel they cannot do without thei *symptom*, that they have to *hold on* to it. Interpreting the pleasure linked to th symptom as the sole motive here would be too superficial. The reason why the often clutch so ferociously to the symptom, as if clinging to a rescue line, is tha this is their only way of feeling alive, their only refuge and chance for stabiliza tion. This attitude is often combined with ego-syntonic symptom coping; th symptom can be reconciled with the self-image, induces no feelings of sham or guilt and is occasionally stylized into an ideology, for example by pedo philes. Patients who continue to be dependent on their symptom often provok the therapist into dreaming up unrealistic therapy goals which go far beyon the patient's abilities. In these cases it is vital that therapy does not focus solel on removing the symptom; instead, the limits of therapy should be accepte and the priority should, for instance, be to enable the patient to learn to contr his symptom better.

So far we have only outlined special aspects of the general framework and o the initial therapeutic contact which present problems. Any pressure from ou side which brought these patients to therapy also creates a chance for therap (see also Goudsmit and Reicher 1980; Petri 1980; Bronisch 1983). A form structure is offered which makes it difficult for the patient to do the obviou avoid facing up to his overall dilemma and resort to acting it out. The initi contacts, to which the patient is more or less forced, decide whether the form framework will gain substance and a therapeutic relationship will develop.

4.2.3 Revising the Concept of Motivation

We have described in detail the patients' and the therapist's problems and th special features of their initial situation in order to elucidate and explain ou conclusion: it is imperative to revise the traditional concept of motivation, least for patients with sexually deviant behaviour. We found a great variety c motives which lead patients to therapy; all must be taken into account and re ognized as legitimate. There is no scale for judging the validity of motives; a d vision into "inner" and "outer", "real" and "unreal" motivation does no justic to the patient's problems. Besides, there are many different reasons why a pa tient resists therapy, is sceptical or anxious; these should also be respected, taken seriously and understood.

It is vital to revise the motivation model for the following reason: as we mentioned, a small number of patients (in our case: about one fifth to a quarter) are motivated for therapy, in the traditional sense, right from the start. There is a danger of devoting therapy exclusively to this group because it is less tiresome and does not require the therapist to adjust his approach. If patients are selected according to their education, insight into their problem and introspective ability one throws away the chance of making psychotherapy available to a wider range of patients; those who do not fulfill these classical criteria are abandoned too quickly. Motivation for therapy also means challenging the patient to be able to and to want to anticipate and accept the psychotherapist's offer of a relationship and therapy, i.e. her/his understanding of psychotherapy. Initially this ability will be missing in many of the patients. Although inner willingness is important, and a problem we by no means underestimate, one cannot help thinking that "motivation for therapy" is often used as a kind of weapon with which patients can be got rid of with a clear conscience.

Understanding that one has to dispense with the concept of motivation was a *result* of our work, and not a premise. This key problem preoccupied us during our entire project. We assessed the patients against variables and categories taken from the motivation model. We therefore included the variable distress and found that 85% were affected by it, 40% extremely so. It was usually manifested in a diffuse unease, a helplessness difficult to articulate and was often not linked to the sexual symptom at all. We noticed that in spite of this distress motivation, in the sense of willingness to actively help deal with the inner problem, was far less common. At the same time we discovered that therapy was possible with patients who had no such motivation. We concluded from this at first that, on the one hand, we had perhaps defined the concept of motivation too narrowly. In the course of the project and with growing therapeutic experience we found that we retrospectively rated the patients' initial motivation as having been better. On the other hand, we had thought secondary motivation, in the sense described, could be gradually achieved during the therapeutic process. Just how questionable the concept of motivation in itself is was something we only realized when the patients and the therapeutic process were assessed after therapy by a rater group. There proved to be another level, quite separate from motivation, on which one could gauge the chances for therapy.

This other level is the *therapeutic relationship*. The *problem of motivation* dissolves or leads into an *interaction problem*. In assessing and evaluating the therapies which had an effect and were successful, we found that the patient-therapist relationship was the decisive driving force, even when there was no motivation in the above sense of a willingness to work actively on dealing with the inner problem. We shall describe how the therapeutic process developed in more detail in Sect. 4.3.

The fact that the motivation problem merges into the relationship problem has one important *practical consequence*: the standard psychotherapeutic practice of assessing motivation in a patient by initially ascribing him this particular characteristic, and viewing this as a prerequisite for therapy or success, is of no use here. It does not even succeed when one scales down the motivation requirements and reduces them, for instance, to willingness to reliably keep appointments, as this kind of reliability can only be the result of a growing trust in the therapist. Even in initial interviews assessing the potential for a relationship is only possible within limits. The range of therapeutic opportunities with these patients can only be fathomed by the therapist showing himself completely prepared to embark on therapy in spite of all the impeding factors.

4.3 The Therapist-Patient Relationship

In the previous section we saw how the initial therapist-patient contact is affected by special circumstances prior to therapy and the way patient and therapist deal with them, on the one hand, and patient pathology, on the other. Seen in this light, it became evident that the concept of therapy motivation had to be revised and that motivation merged into in the problem of the therapeutic relationship.

Although it is stressing the obvious to view the therapeutic relationship as the pivotal point of therapy, this point has only recently been discussed in behaviour therapy literature and has in particular been neglected in therapy for sexual delinquents: focussing on the conspicuous deviant symptom tempts one to isolate it and make the patient the object of treatment and not the subject (see Sect. 1.3.1). We have repeatedly described in previous sections how closely the symptom is interwoven with a patient's personality and his abilities to cope with life. We shall now describe the links revealed in the therapeutic relationship.

Data from the evaluation by the rater group based on the inductively developed category system (see p. 22) form the first basis for description and analysis of the therapeutic relationship Altogether 17 variables were included in data analysis: 8 variables which describe the patient's behaviour and emotional reaction to therapy and the therapist; 9 variables which describe the behaviour and reaction of the therapist to the patient.

In the *first step* all the therapies were evaluated using these variables.

In the *second step* correlation analysis was used to relate the relationship variables to one another and to the variables of the patient's personality structure and problem. Factor analysis was used to analyse the structure of the therapeutic relationship, mean comparison and correlation statistics to analyse the correlation with other patient variables. We are aware that this statistical approach does not enable one to trace the subtle interactions and developmental changes in the course of therapy. However, it gave us a framework within which the processes in the therapeutic relationship could be described.

4.3.1 Factors in the Therapeutic Relationship

Patient and therapist variables were factor analysed separately[1] Factors were described with variables that loaded with 0.40 or more.

Patient Factors

1. *"Childlike submission" vs. "distance"* (36% of total variance; 63.8% explained variance)

Variables:
- Submission/overadapting/letting things happen to oneself (0.81)
- Childlike dependency (0.76)
- Emphasizing helplessness and weakness (-0.54)
- Emphasizing strength and independence (-0.60)
- Open rejection of relationship (-0.46)

2. "Active cooperation" vs. "refusal" (21.3% of total variance, 36.2% of explained variance)

Variables:
- Willingness to cooperate actively (0.95)
- Indirect rejection of relationship (e.g. withdrawal, pseudo-intimacy, playing a role, reducing therapist to a function) (-0.64)

Therapist Factors

1. *"Showing emotional interest in patient" vs. "keeping emotional distance"* (33.5% of total variance, 68.2% of explained variance)

Variables:
- Interest in the patient (0.66)
- Sympathy for the patient (0.58)
- Keeping emotional distance to patient (-0.69)
- Annoyance at patient (-0.60)
- Helplessness with patient (-0.55)

2. *"Overeagerness and control"* (19.3% of total variance, 31.8% of explained variance)

Variables:
- Therapist overinvolved (0.69)
- Unrealistic assessment of patient by therapist (0.63)
- Control of patient by therapist (0.55)

These four factors in the therapist-patient relationship will be used as new numerical variables below. Our method here is analogous to our factor analysis of coping strategies (see p. 52).

The degree to which therapy was influenced by emotions and behaviour patterns bundled in these factors is shown in Table 8.[2]

---

[1] Principal axis factor analysis with iteration: number of extracted factors according to criterion eigenvalue is <1; Varimax rotation; an experimental oblique rotation produced an analogous factor structure.

[2] Distribution of values was transformed back to the scale: not present, present, markedly present.

From the *patient's angle*, the relationship is more strongly influenced by "childlike submission" than by "distance". The number of patients who refused to cooperate is strikingly high; active cooperation was rare by comparison. Neither patient factor correlates with the other.

Table 8. Weight of factors in therapist-patient relationship

Patient variable factors	n[a]	Pronounced %	Evident %	Not evident %	Evident %	Pronounced %	
1. Childlike submission	57	25	29	24	10	12	vs. reserve
2. Active cooperation	58	2	21	26	16	35	vs. refusal
Therapist variable factors	**n*ea**	**Pronounced**	**Evident**	**Not evident**	**Evident**	**Pronounced**	
1. Emotional interest in patient	59	44	11	24	12	9	vs. keeping emotional distance
2. Overeagerness and control	57	19	36	45	–	–	–

[a] Due to decrease in n, see footnote 3 on p. 128.

Table 9

	Childlike submission vs. distance	Active cooperation vs. refusal
Emotional interest in patient vs. reserve	–	0.57 ($p<1\%$)
Overeagerness and control	–	-0.32 ($p<1\%$)

Seen from the *therapist's angle*, therapy was influenced more by "emotional interest in the pa tient" than by "keeping emotional distance". Although not very pronounced, the emotion and kinds of behaviour combined in the factors "overeagerness and control" did play a role i a large number of therapies. Both factors correlate with each other ($r=-0.39$, $p<1\%$): greate emotional reserve on the therapist's part was significantly more frequently combined witl overeagerness and control.

The correlations between patient and therapist variable factors are shown in Table 9.

The first factor ("childlike submission" vs. "distance"), which explains most of the variance does not correlate with either of the therapist factors. By contrast, the second factor ("activ cooperation" vs. "refusal") correlates with both therapist factors: a stronger, hidden reserve o the patient's part was significantly often combined particularly with the therapist's emotiona distance, but also with overeagerness and control.

4.3.2 First Patient Factor: "Childlike Submission" vs. "Keeping One's Distance"

When interpreted, the two poles of this factor represent two opposite ways of dealing with the same kind of problem: there is a disturbance in the development of autonomy. More specifically, we are faced with two pathological relationship patterns:

First, there are patients with clinging mothers who obstruct autonomy and give no or little support to a healthy desire to become self-reliant. Regressive symbiotic desires persist in later relationships with a tendency to submit and cling; aggressive emotions often of a destructive nature are vigorously warded off.

Second, there are patients who were left alone too early as children, had to fend for themselves and were unable to grow up with the trusting feeling of being safe, sheltered and protected. To avoid experiencing a revival of previous disappointments, which they unconsciously anticipate when forming any relationship, these patients constantly have to prove their self-reliance and independence of the environment and their contemporaries; they are suspicious of and avoid relationships and adopt a pseudo-autonomy with which they can hold their desires for dependency in check. This leads to even greater withdrawal, a sign of a deep-rooted mistrust. This problem in relationships also plays an important role in the therapeutic process.

The one pole ("childlike submission", pronounced in a quarter of the patients - see Table 8) is a striking and typical relationship pattern although it can be variously accented: while some patients captivate the therapist with their childlike and disarming charm, are likable, nonaggressive and allow themselves to be easily led, others appear as helpless and passive as a small child, and yet others submit to the therapist in a masochistic manner and avoid having any opinion of their own.

These different shades of childlike submission have one feature in common: delegating responsibility to the therapist. The difficulty is that these patients, with their meagre ability to assert themselves and their unwillingness to face any conflict, try to withdraw from constructive discussion in therapy. Accordingly the therapist sees no trace of aggression, or notices a fluctuating aggression in the countertransference, although it is not really tangible here either.

We have chosen two examples for the "childlike submission" factor; the first illustrates amiable, boyish affection, the second more the regressive, infantile aspects.

Case 6 (previous history: see p. 44)

Outpatient therapy with a female therapist lasted 3 years with long intermissions. At the start of therapy the patient was unemployed and saw no prospects of finding a job. His exhibitionism was a particularly pressing problem. His desolate situation, combined with a confiding manner and a childlike charm, awakened the therapist's empathy, sympathy and maternal feelings. His impressive skills in adapting and orienting to others' expectations determined his behaviour. He actually insisted on being mothered by the therapist, let her lead and steer him and handed over all responsibility for himself to her. Nevertheless his behaviour contained elements of an indirect resistance and refusal: he was not very reliable in keeping appointments, usually only came to therapy when in difficulty, emphasizing how helpless and lacking in support he was. Basically he refused to face up to himself; it seemed almost impossible to confront him with conflicts and problems. He was evasive and directed attention again and again to the surrounding situation and circumstances. For him the therapist had a protective maternal function. She reacted to his unreliableness by developing ways of controlling him.

Therapy focussed on symptom control; the patient cooperated like a "good boy". In coping with ongoing conflicts such as acute marital crises and unemployment he was offered help; the attempt to deal with his partner problems failed early on because neither he nor his wife was basically interested. The patient rewarded the therapist by continually reassuring her how good therapy was for him, how much it helped him. It was impossible to find out what he really felt.

During therapy he relapsed twice; these relapses – and in fact any difficulty – were the excuse for him to return to the therapist. It seemed as though the therapist concealed her aggressive feelings to maintain a harmonious relationship. Therapy was marked by a lack of conflict and friendly noncommitment although the patient did gradually manage to control his symptom better. He stabilized further after retraining and finding a job and when his wife became pregnant. His first reaction to her pregnancy was anxiety, but he was full of pride when the child arrived. The marriage improved after the birth.

At *follow-up* 3½ years after therapy he reported no longer having any exhibitionist desires. At the time of writing, 3 years after the last follow-up, the patient has not called again although he usually returns to us immediately after a relapse. It is only to be hoped that his problem is now less acute.

In summary the symptom was reduced during therapy, certainly also because his social situation improved; the patient's central problem remained however unaffected. Essentially his relationship to the therapist repeated the pathological interaction pattern, i.e. excluding the patient's anxieties and lack of trust concealed behind his amiability.

Case 5 (previous history: see p. 42)

Therapy lasted 2 years with 68 sessions at weekly, towards the end at fortnightly intervals. Except for an unsettled beginning appointments were reliably kept.

His reaction to imprisonment (cardiac neurosis symptoms) demonstrated how closely the patient was attached to his mother. The initial therapeutic contacts were overshadowed by the patient's acute heart complaints which he described in dramatic terms and were combined with states of anxiety, insomnia and medication abuse.

The acuteness of these disorders at first impeded any structuring of therapy and dominated the initial phase in which the (female) therapist was confused by the patient's helplessness and panic; the latter had his wife or mother bring him to the appointments. Although the therapist felt sorry for him and developed maternal feelings, she also felt annoyed because he blamed his environment for his suffering. He delegated all responsibility to her; she was supposed to know what was right; he wanted to place himself entirely in her hands. The therapist's attempts to talk about the offences failed. The patient's fear dominated the situation and the therapist failed to understand its significance sufficiently. As a consequence he did not feel understood or in good hands, but experienced therapy as exacting and demanding and acted evasively by persisting in a regressive, infantile helplessness. The therapist reacted more and more by making suggestions and expecting him to take over responsibility for himself; the first sessions thus turned full circle with no progress made. The situation became calmer once she stopped making demands on him, offered herself as an interested and patient listener and showed sympathetic interest in his experience in prison, which still troubled him very much. The sessions were then dominated by current problems, particularly his wife's wish to leave him which reactivated powerful anxieties. In the process of this separation he started clinging to the therapist who then began to discuss this problem: his anxiety, lack of trust, insecurity, all feelings concealed behind his childlike, submissive stance. The relationship to the therapist gradually gave him so much security that he could slightly modify his regressive attitude: he came to therapy alone, the cardiac neurosis symptom was no longer acute. During these first steps towards more adult behaviour, he was nonetheless irritable and was easily overstrained. These first improvements were maintained during the second year of treatment and he was able to accept a more personal approach. He started thinking about his offence and, for the first time, felt guilty. He talked about how disappointed he had been by women, but would not permit any discussion of his relationship to his mother.

Treatment was discontinued at the patient's request.

In *follow-up sessions* 1 year after therapy the patient made a rather phlegmatic, subdepressive impression. He had put on weight. He said he hardly had any sexual desires any more. He had not committed another sexual offence. All in all, his perspective on life was uncertain; after being in prison he had failed to find a new job. Private contacts were confined to his family home; he still had a very close relationship to his mother.

In summary, treatment helped the patient to cope with a crisis caused by a 2½ year prison sentence and an ensuing acute regression. Moreover, the patient made some progress towards maturity in as much as the therapeutic relationship taught him to see his life more realistically and, by giving up projection, accept that he was responsible for his own fortune. However, he did not manage to make active use of the experiences he had gathered in therapy. Deviant actingout and the associated protest against dependency on his mother were exchanged for subdepressive resignation. We are not sure how this patient will develop further.

The other pole of the factor, keeping one's distance (pronounced in 12% of patients, see Table 8) is a relationship pattern which has an important protective function for the patients: they emphasize their selfreliance to the therapist because they are afraid of dependency. Many say they fear something happening against their will and arm themselves against this. Feelings are seen as a sign of weakness. Despite this superficially negative attitude, which these patients use to try to protect themselves from being spurned and disappointed, a subconscious desire for intimacy and acceptance shines through in many of them, even though they are unable to see it themselves, or at least cannot admit it.

For the therapist this hidden longing for intimacy is often scarcely visible as it is smothered by the patient's fear. If the therapist insists too soon on the patient relinquishing this reserved attitude, the danger is the patient will discontinue therapy.[3] If, on the other hand, the therapist respects the patient's need repeatedly to reassure himself of his independence, there is a chance that a therapeutic relationship may nonetheless develop.

Case 17 (Previous history: see p. 72)

Therapy lasted 1½ years with 52 sessions. The patient kept appointments; he was very anxious to "get rid of" his exhibitionism which was an urgent problem. He called it his "only weakness" and was set on avoiding discussion of other problems. He refused to recognize any connection between his symptom and his personality. It was important for him to point out and emphasize his strength, independence and ability to get his own way to the therapist again and again; in doing so he implied he was not prepared to think about why he needed this manly façade.

The *therapist* reacted sympathetically to the at least superficially open and charming patient, but felt impatient because he sensed it was very difficult to reach him. The latter was unable to

[3] The following statistics show that the risk of therapy being broken off is very high, particularly here: in therapy dropouts relationship structures seeking dependency are significantly less frequent ($p < 1\%$).

question the tediously erected defence against his fear of being a basically weak, small and inadequate man. The therapeutic situation was an insult, as he was unable to define himself as someone who had needs and weaknesses and was highly vulnerable. He remained wary and kept his distance.

Therapy focussed on two aspects: first, and typical for the first phase, the therapist went along with the patient's way of viewing the symptom as an isolated problem. Behaviourist symptom control methods were used at first to support the patient's willingness for therapy. In the second phase, the therapist carefully started discussing problem areas such as family conflicts, his vulnerability, his tendency to have impulsive aggressive outbursts and to numb himself with alcohol, and the link between these problems and the exhibitionist symptom. This succeeded gradually as a good emotional relationship developed and the patient became able to get more involved - as it were, against his will. His reactions to being confronted with his problem were typical: after relaxing his rigid control in one session and questioning himself, in the next session he began by describing in detail how successful and strong he was at work in an effort to impress the therapist with his stamina and virility. After this ritual of reassuring himself of his independence and strength, he was able to open up a little, although he was not really able to give up his reserve.

In the *course of therapy* the symptom became much less acute. The patient was at least partially willing to relativize his rigid masculine ideal and to see his aggressive defence against conflicts with his wife not only as a sign of strength, but also as a way of evading a discussion. He was able to control his alcohol consumption very much better. At least occasionally he understood that feelings of powerlessness and weakness underlay his persistent demonstration of how strong and independent he was.

These incipient changes remained very unstable. Unfortunately therapy was discontinued because the therapist left us. This was a great disappointment to the patient, who was not prepared to adjust to another therapist. When the therapist announced he was leaving, he closed up again and demanded anti-androgen medication; in so doing he retreated to his initial view that his desire to expose himself was an isolated problem. As it later turned out, a relapse occurred at the time therapy was discontinued.

The factor "childlike submission" vs. "keeping one's distance" corresponds to the main factor in the patients' coping strategies "avoiding intimacy" vs. "dependency in relationships" (see p. 56). The factors correlate highly. [4] "Childlike submission" in therapy is, however, very much more frequent than "dependency in relationships". This is due to the nature of therapeutic contact: first, the power is unevenly divided; second, the therapist's helper role makes it easier for the patient to act exactly as he feels, to be weak, helpless and dependent, rather than to protect or hide himself or to make himself less vulnerable.

A correlation was found between this patient factor in the therapeutic relationship and the patients in cluster 2 (see p. 69): the patients in cluster 2 show the greatest tendency to deviate from the overall mean value towards "childlike submission". These patients are typically depressive and have a very negative self-image and potency disorders, tend to become dependent and let themselves be supported by others. The patients in cluster 5 (see p. 73) on the other hand, who are severely disturbed social outsiders, usually incapable of relating

[4] The calculated product-moment correlation coefficient $r = 0.61$ does not show the exact height of the correlation since the distribution of the patients in the factors differs from the normal distribution.

to others and very aggressive, show a deviation away from the overall mean towards the other pole, "keeping one's distance".

The patient factor "childlike submission" vs. "keeping one's distance" is connected with a fundamental problem these patients have in relating to others which is mirrored and re-enacted in the therapeutic situation. Interestingly enough, no statistical correlation could be found between this patient factor and the two therapist factors which describe the therapist's emotional attitude. This may be because the therapist takes a more diagnostic view of the patient's difficulties in relating to others and sees it as a symptom.

4.3.3 The Second Patient Factor: "Active Cooperation" vs. "Refusal"

Whilst the first patient factor describes patients' basic problems in relating at all, the second - "active cooperation" vs. "refusal" - describes more the concrete interaction in the therapy session and is concerned much more directly with the patient's attitudes to and behaviour in therapy, i.e. it includes the therapist as a person who reacts emotionally to the patient's attitude and behaviour. There are therefore characteristic correlations between this patient factor and the two therapist factors. We should like to describe these interaction dynamics, as far as they statistically correspond to the patient and therapist factors, in more detail by outlining the factors for therapist variables.

One pole of this patient factor, *"active cooperation"*, is characterized by a marked interest in therapy and reliability in keeping appointments. The patients on their own initiative introduce topics or material for the therapy, accept supportive interventions, cooperate in behaviour therapy exercises, try to confront and interprete their situation, look for new aspects in their emotional reactions in therapy, etc. There is a significant correlation with certain initial characteristics such as inhibited aggression, tendency towards depression, no severe disturbance, fairly good social integration ($p < 1\%$). Their problems are not as pronounced, but similar to those of patients described in cluster 1 (psychically more stable, socially integrated patient group) and cluster 2 (depressive patient group). In the section on motivation we pointed out that some of these patients (one fifth to a quarter) were motivated for therapy right from the start; "active cooperation" was also seen in 25%, and the groups seem to be more or less identical. There is a close correlation between the second patient factor and the *first therapist factor* ($r = 0.57$): "active cooperation" by a patient arouses emotional involvement in the therapist, combined with acceptance, sympathy and interest in the patient.

Case 15 (Previous history: see p. 68)

As the patient lived in southern Germany a 6-week inpatient therapy with daily sessions was organized. The patient paid the hospital expenses himself. He had not relapsed since being charged 6 months prior to therapy. Therapy was conducted by a male therapist. The patient's initial fears in therapy led to an interaction pattern which proved to be typical for him: in the first sessions his flow of words was difficult to interrupt at all and the therapist was unable to recognize what was personally important to the patient. On the one hand, this characteristic behaviour served to meet what he assumed to be the therapist's requirements and to court his good will; his monologizing was, on the other hand, a way of preventing interference in order to maintain his independence in the sessions. With growing mutual familiarity he was able to calm down and listen attentively, and tried to piece together the psychological situation for himself. The sessions centred on his anxiety in facing up to conflicts and his fear of losing out in discussions. The fear of feeling inferior to the therapist shone clearly through his strenuously amiable courting of him.

The patient at first avoided talking about his sexuality and desire to expose himself. Underlying this was an enormous lack of self-confidence in himself as a man with male potency which he imagined would destroy any harmonious relationship. This was the patient's first opportunity to talk "man to man" about the fears he associated with sexuality and to see them in a wider context. In retrospect it became clear that he had been deeply upset about physical changes during puberty when his first desires to expose himself emerged.

In the last phase of therapy he was able to understand that his numerous leisure activities served to distract him from his inferiority feelings toward his wife. He expressed the wish to deal with this in couple therapy with his wife after being discharged.

After therapy the patient kept in contact with the therapist on his own initiative. No relapse has yet occurred during the 2 years of follow-up.

In summary, the patient was treated for psychosexual maturation deficits in the oedipal phase, whereas his ego development was relatively "healthy". During this short, intensive therapy it was important both to understand the meaning behind the symptom as the aftermath of childhood anxieties and also to succeed in forming a good, cooperative atmosphere in which the patient, despite his anxieties about his masculinity, could reveal his doubts and fears to a man.

The second pole of this factor, "refusal", covers a characteristic and frequent attitude in these patients during therapy: reserve, restraint, apprehensiveness, keeping a sceptical distance. This attempt to keep the therapist at arm's length is not, however, openly expressed; it takes a great variety of forms. This stance could be observed in half of the patients and was pronounced in one third. There is a correlation with the following patient variables: pronounced personality disturbance ($p < 1\%$), social outsider ($p < 5\%$), and with the coping strategies "avoiding intimacy" ($r = 0.30$) and "manipulative, indirect aggression" ($r = 0.48$).

The frequency of these attitudes can only partly be attributed to the patient's problem and no doubt has something to do with the objective conditions at the start of therapy, described in the last section, which initially arouse the patients' suspicions.

There are *various accentuations* within this factor which have a major influence on the therapeutic process:

"Refusal" may describe only one aspect of the relationship pattern. Although the therapist may experience that his empathy is answered by the patient withdrawing and refusing to commit himself, this reserve and constraint – often concealed beneath a superficial openness and willingness to cooperate – are nonetheless intermingled with a secret longing to be totally accepted. Both his anxiety about being questioned and the desire to be accepted with all his shortcomings are reflected in the patient's *ambivalence toward the therapist.* As long as the therapist is aware of this ambivalence and can sense the patient's desire for a relationship despite his apparent lack of interest, he is more likely to succeed in understanding the patient's adamant attitude as a defence strategy, as a partial, stabilizing retreat and to respond warmheartedly in the sense of the one pole in the first therapist factor. Accordingly, the therapeutic attitude in this pole ("emotional interest in the patient") is very much more frequent (over half the cases) than the "active cooperation" pole in the patient factor.

Case 13 (previous history: see p. 62)

Therapy lasted 48 sessions over 1½ years. The patient's tendency to withdraw from others, to keep a safe distance, to intellectualize problems and his willingness to adapt well also shaped the therapist-patient relationship at first: although reliable in keeping appointments, he remained sceptical and taciturn, said little about himself, was very ashamed of his exhibitionism and was intent on keeping the relationship neutral. He did not want to risk committing himself. He dealt with his problems like mental puzzles which had to be solved and was clearly afraid of being laughed at by the therapist.

The therapist handled him very carefully, at first respected his desire to keep a distance, stayed in the background and took his deep embarrassment and fear of showing his shortcomings into account.

The therapy threatened to stagnate into a sober, ritualized game, but this was decisively interrupted by a court hearing to which the therapist also went, although not as an expert witness. The patient saw the hearing as a way of testing whether the therapist's interest in him was genuine, whether he would stand by him and not abandon him. Afterwards he was more approachable, gradually began talking about himself and relaxing slightly. A discussion of the symptom began in which his problem was placed in a context which helped him to understand that exposing himself was a way of escaping from his sense of emptiness and loneliness.

The main focus of therapy was the therapist-patient interaction. The most important result for the patient seemed to be his ability to confide in someone without being denigrated. He started facing up to confrontations and interpretations without immediately having to "parry". Making use of this good relationship, the therapist introduced some symptom control techniques and instructions on how to deal with other people. This proved effective as these structured tasks coincided with the patient's basic view that his inner problems were tasks to be solved pragmatically.

At the end of therapy the patient no longer felt quite as much at the mercy of his exhibitionist impulses. He was now better able to tackle problems and assert himself at work. He was no longer so reticent and cautiously began to approach other people. Follow-up results are not yet available.

In summary, treatment was a corrective emotional experience: contrary to his own expectations, the patient felt he was taken seriously by the therapist, despite his shortcomings and mistakes. A growing understanding of his symptoms reduced his feelings of shame and guilt and strengthened his self-confidence, and this helped him gradually to come out of his shell. This was an important prerequisite for dispensing with the symptom which we considered to be a substitute for relationships, among other things.

"Refusal" can, however, be *more obvious and pronounced* and may take different forms: a patient can conceal his refusal behind pseudo-intimacy or behind a façade. The therapist increasingly senses that he is not getting through to the patient at all with his offer of a relationship. Alternatively, therapeutic efforts merely lead to pseudo-therapy because the patient sees the therapist as a representative of the institution "therapy as punishment" and tries to use the therapist for his own objectives. A few patients showed a remarkable ability to fulfill the requirements in the court order by only getting involved enough for the therapist to keep hoping that therapy might make some sense after all; nevertheless they withdrew again by skipping therapy sessions or playing down conflicts and difficulties. Behind this kind of *functionalizing refusal* lies suspicion and fear. The therapist is perceived as the representative or henchman of the authorities intent on retribution, as an opponent difficult to grapple with, against whom one has to defend oneself; mistrust and tactical behaviour seem best if one is to protect one's own interest and keep out of harm's way. Mistrust is mixed with fear because the patient is confronted with a situation in which something is meant to happen to him and this means that the symptom he feels protects him is going to be "done away with".

It was obviously much more difficult for therapists to deal with this kind of relationship, as typified in the second patient factor ("refusal"), than with "keeping one's distance", the first patient factor. The results of factor analysis showed two characteristic *forms of therapist reaction*:

1. The therapist feels overwhelmed and helpless when the patient acts out his symptom, feels exploited by him and is angry with the patient; a positive relationship and feelings such as sympathy and interest refuse to evolve. The therapist escapes by generating his own *emotional distance*. This is the second pole of the first therapist factor, which was more or less pronounced in one fifth of therapies. We found a correlation with patients in cluster 5 (the group of severely disturbed, social outsiders), i.e. with patients who we described as aggressive, for the most part incapable of relating to others, socially isolated and who had mostly committed violent sexual offences.

Case 11 (previous history: see p. 58)

After missing several appointments the patient seemed depressive, accusatory, moody and taciturn in the first session. The therapist felt faced with a chaotic situation and did not know where to start. In supervision we considered taking this patient into a group, not without some doubt as to whether this might be too demanding on him. He remained evasive in the group and after a few sessions failed to reappear. He contacted the therapist again when acute crises occurred. Therapy proved impossible because he failed to keep appointments. He came when he felt bad, threatened to commit suicide, was reproachful and warded off any discussion about himself, his life and his symptom (homosexual pedophilia). A personal relationship to the therapist did not develop; the patient saw him merely as an impersonal point of contact. A change of therapist met with scarcely any reaction either. The atmosphere improved somewhat after the therapist gave up the idea of continuous therapy with the patient and accepted his rather more anonymous role. The therapist no longer felt as helpless or angry but became less involved and no longer felt under pressure. Although the patient showed no continuous development, the therapeutic contacts over the last 5 years seem to have given the patient a certain amount of stability in his chaotic life.

To summarize, it was impossible to help this patient make any steps towards maturity as he used therapy exclusively as a means to support his illusionistic, regressive wishes. It is extremely doubtful whether the patient's functionalizing, parasitical adherence to the Department of Sex Research can act as an effective rescue line in the long run as he avoids commitments and any confrontation with reality.

2. Another kind of reaction on the therapist's part is the second therapist factor "overeagerness and control". We consider this to be an important and characteristic reaction and attitude in some therapies ("overeagerness and control" was pronounced in one fifth of the therapies; elements of this reaction were demonstrable in one third; see Table 8). In this factor the therapist's behaviour is marked less by empathy, sympathy and understanding for the patient than by the assumption that he/she is responsible for the patient's fate. The therapist judges the patient's chances unrealistically, in particular by overestimating his capacity for relating to others. The therapist would like to "save" the patient at all costs; the patient's precarious social situation caused by his deviancy becomes a threat to the therapist which the latter has difficulty tolerating. It can happen that the therapist seeks refuge in indiscriminate therapeutic activity without ever dealing with the reasons for the patient's adamancy. The therapist then runs the risk of becoming a powerful authority exerting control over the patient without noticing that this asymmetry in the relationship results in a reinforcement of the refusal behaviour and causes the patient, who feels powerless, to regress to passivity and dependency. The patient as he truly is fades in significance compared with the therapist's compulsive urge to do something for him.

Our interpretation of this factor, which is frequently found in directive, structuring therapy, should not be taken to mean that this is always and inevitably a senseless or false therapeutic attitude. Activity, structuring and guidance can give both therapist and patient a framework which can aid therapy (see Case 9, p. 126). The therapist's feeling that he is not reaching the withdrawn patient frequently evokes the wish to structure the therapeutic situation even more, in order to get a grip on the patient whose ambiguity signals an emotional need despite his refusal.

This therapeutic approach is potentially dangerous. When faced with helplessness and anger, the wish to structure tempts one to use therapeutic programmes and methods as a means of exerting power. A behaviour therapy approach then tempts the therapist to counter the patient's ambiguity with a clear-cut plan. The patient's inability to give up his symptom, which is interpreted as indecision, is confronted with the decisiveness of symptom control. The patient's skill in functionalizing relationships comes up against the power tool of a hierarchical training programme for socially adequate behaviour. The therapist then runs the risk of relapsing into activity for its own sake or turning therapy into a covert power struggle.

Case 7 (previous history, see p. 46)

The patient had recently felt that he was unable to control his impulse to expose himself any longer and since then had been running from therapist to therapist, sometimes entertaining several at once. Not his symptom, but its effects were his problem. The interaction always had the same pattern: in the first few sessions he demonstrated how splendid he was, attempted to impress the listener with his fantastic life story, his potency and success with women; all this was at first a challenge to the therapist. Whenever his self-aggrandisement was questioned he stayed away and went to the next therapist to whom he complained about the previous therapists, but then acted in the same manner again.

The first phase of treatment (30 sessions) was carried out by a female therapist. The patient insisted on restricting treatment to his work and learning problems; he did not want to touch on the sexual problems. The therapist acquiesced at first in the hope that she could thereby gain access to his problems. This attempt failed because the patient constantly withdrew and ignored plans. He was incapable of accepting anything from the therapist, as this would have undermined his grandiose idea of himself. He soon began making sexual approaches to the therapist, sexualizing this contact as well, and did not return once this attempt failed.

A year later he returned and was assigned to a male therapist. This time the patient defined symptom control as the focus of therapy; it was typical of him to dictate the terms. He exerted a blackmailing pressure by threatening to seek stereotactic brain surgery and let us know that we were responsible for his fate. The patient seemed to be both helpless and overpowering; the therapist felt partly ineffectual and partly assumed the responsibility handed over to him by the patient by starting a control programme. A sadomasochistic relationship pattern developed which precluded empathy and provoked aggressive countertransference emotions. These in turn gave the therapist a bad conscience and he turned to the team for long discussions on how to proceed in therapy. This was the only patient who provoked us into considering using aversive methods. This therapeutic experiment proved senseless. We came to realize that this method was an expression of our own sadistic impulses in the countertransference, triggered by our helplessness when faced with our inability to reach the patient.

Two years later the patient returned for a medical report. In the meantime he had been discovered exposing himself. A 90-page report was written; in the trial the patient was cleared of the charges. He was obviously able to impress his "uniqueness" on the court and the expert.

To summarize, given this patient's severe personality disorders it proved impossible to establish a therapeutic relationship which could have formed the basis for a joint effort. Experience with other patients has also shown us that patients whose perversion is embedded in a severe narcissistic character pathology are for the most part impervious to psychotherapy.

4.4 The Therapeutic Approach

4.4.1 Planning Therapy: Finding a Therapeutic Gestalt

Behind the repeated call for a special psychotherapeutic "treatment programme" for sex offenders has always been the assumption that these patients essentially all suffer from the same problems. This is clearly shown in early attempts by behaviour therapists to develop a *one-dimensional,* usually symptom-focussed therapeutic procedure for standard "use". This procedure is then justified by regarding sexual arousability via deviant stimuli as a phenomenon which does not require further examination. Alternatively specific anxieties (such as fears of failure in a heterosexual encounter or behaviour deficits such as problems in relating to others) which are frequently linked to sexual deviancy, are picked out and regarded as the cause of the deviancy. This one-dimensional approach has hardly any backing in today's behaviour therapy literature. Our results on the structure and psychodynamics of our patients also refute any such assumption of homogeneity.

More recent *multi-dimensional* behaviour therapy approaches take account of the wide range of disturbances. Attention is focussed on the whole range of the patient's symptoms; several areas of disturbance are singled out in order to assign special therapeutic techniques to them. This supposedly enables the therapists to adapt the therapeutic procedure better to a patient's individual problems (see Sect. 1.3.1). The treatment programme is no longer a one-dimensional model, but a kind of construction set: in each patient various problem areas are picked out and the appropriate therapy programme is chosen. This approach aims at choosing the best procedure out of a selection of prefabricated therapeutic programmes.

This multi-dimensional approach also has serious disadvantages as it is merely a cumulative combination of ready-to-use methods. Just as learning theory has no elaborated theory of sexual perversion, these therapeutic approaches dispense with attempting to understand a patient's individual (sexual) symptoms in the course of therapy. It is, however, hard to conceive how one can find a meaningful focus for therapy without *psychodynamic insight*. Applying prefabricated programmes to patients leads to a startling contrast between impressive success rates with some patients and gross failure with others, without any understanding of why this is so.

Another serious shortcoming is that this concept completely neglects the *therapeutic relationship* and its dynamics during therapy. It is then usually subsumed under intervening variable. What is overlooked is that the therapeutic relationship not only determines what is feasible and what is not, but also that this relationship and its dynamics form a key component of therapy.

The final consequence of the meanwhile common criticism of this kind of therapy and research is to *reject* the concept of designing prefabricated *treatment programmes* which can be taught from an instruction manual. The idea that programmes and methods can be applied to everyone presupposes patient uniformity; otherwise it would be illogical.

Dispensing with programmes, however, certainly does not mean dispensing with any kind of therapy planning or systematic and structured procedure. Nor does it mean that we refuse to use *deliberately chosen* and practical behaviour therapy instructions and methods. Deliberately chosen means asking, analysing and pinpointing the implications of such interventions for the therapist-patient relationship and their effects on the patient's psychodynamics.

In programmatic terms, we introduce the *concept of an evolving, open therapeutic gestalt* as against the concept of a multi-dimensional mosaic of treatment strategies.

The therapist's first concern - which is also his ultimate aim in coming to understand the patient - is to identify what the symptom "says" and what it "means". The true answer to these questions can only be found after a concept for understanding the patient, a gestalt of the patient, has been worked out. Working towards the gestalt of the patient is closely interlinked with developing a therapeutic gestalt; each is a reflection of the other. Conceived in this light, therapy planning orients directly and closely on the patient's problem. If the therapist can grasp the underlying framework, the gestalt behind the patient's actions, she/he can then intervene with appropriately flexible and selected methods. This means that the gestalt has a systematizing effect on the therapeutic procedure.

We should now like to continue this line of thought by giving examples. For reasons of clarity, we shall describe the process of therapy planning as a *heuris-*

tic search process in which we distinguish six aspects. This heuristic model should be seen as an overall framework and not as a replication of the real chronology of the therapeutic process.

1. All these patients have *sexually deviant symptoms* which have a stabilizing function in their psychic organization. Their dependency on this kind of stabilization varies according to the intensity of the disturbance and the availability of other forms of compensation. This is where *an understanding* of the patient begins and is also the first step in the heuristic search process. The usually complex meanings of a particular patient's symptoms and their function can only be pinpointed individually. Like a spotlight, they point out the way to the patient's basic dilemma (see Sect. 3.2).

2. The second step is to discover *the precise problem underlying the perverse symptom*. The type and severity of the disturbance determine the form therapy takes. A patient's problems become visible in the way he both regressively and progressively compensates and defends himself.

3. Patients develop a whole variety of such coping strategies to help them survive socially and psychically despite their problem (see Sect. 3.5). The third step is *analysis of these coping strategies*. Not only do the patient's creative abilities become evident, but also the strategies which, although they help him at least temporarily to stabilize psychically and socially, in the long run leave him permanently labile and easily thrown off balance. In the course of this analysis one comes to recognize which basic problems the patient cannot adequately compensate with the strategies available to him.

4. A patient's coping strategies are reflected in the specific manner in which he acts towards the therapist. The *patient's way of relating* is the fourth aspect. Above all, coping strategies are also *interaction strategies* activated in the *encounter with the therapist* (see Wittmann 1981). Already in the first therapy sessions one can observe how the patient shapes his relationship with the therapist. The patient's behaviour towards the therapist, his usually nonverbal communication of his state of mind and his attempt to structure the relationship reveal the limits of his ability to relate to others and his expectations of the therapist (see Sects. 4.2 and 4.3).

5. The fifth step in this heuristic process is for the therapist to find the right level in the therapeutic encounter so that the patient can enter into a relationship with him. If the key to understanding the patient lies in understanding the meaning and purpose of the perverse symptom, the key to therapy lies in *recognizing which relationship level is feasible*. Ultimately, however, the patient determines the level, depending on the severity of his disturbance and his prevailing coping pattern. As an external point of reference, the therapist can offer the patient a certain, preliminary structure; he can, for example, accept the fact that the patient wants to idealize and obey him, and later gradually insist on more self-reliance. He can keep his distance and so accept the patient's fear of any

kind of intimacy, allowing it to develop gradually in the course of therapy. Whatever the case, the therapist must start by going along with the patient's structuring of the relationship without, however, becoming emotionally biased. This requires a great deal of flexibility on the part of the therapist, which depends in turn on her/his own personality and strategies in life. We shall return to this point later on.

6. Using all these factors as a basis, the sixth step is to take the patient's *current psychosocial situation* into account and finalize the details of therapeutic procedure. The questions here are: whether specific problem areas should be dealt with in therapy and if so, which (for example: sexual symptoms, partnership problems, etc.).

4.4.2 Framework and Focus of Therapy

The heuristic search process oriented directly on the patient's individual problems can sometimes result in very different therapeutic procedures. The difference between each therapeutic gestalt affects not just and not primarily the *thematic foci* in therapy, but also the various *kinds of intervention*. One should remember the difficulties prior to therapy: the patients' lack of trust, their fear of surveillance, their very different social circumstances, personal characteristics and the different ideas about and expectations of therapy. A uniform, prestructured therapeutic concept is clearly inappropriate. Instead, one should carefully work out an opening for therapy for each patient which fits in with his expectations and abilities. As a guide we distinguish between *four levels of therapeutic work and therapeutic approach*: help with everday life, intervention in crises, behaviour therapy for definable problem areas, and interpretation and confrontation. These levels should not be seen too rigidly or as mutually exclusive. They are initial levels of approach to create a basis for therapy acceptable to the patient.

4.4.2.1 Help in Coping with Everyday Life

The *focus* of therapy on this level is mostly help in coping with current and basic everyday problems which often represent an existential threat, especially for patients with few social ties: help with finding or keeping an apartment, work, sorting out financial problems, etc. These social tasks should not be taken on by the therapist himself, but delegated to a probation officer. The therapist can, however, lend support and encouragement, make and maintain contact with the probation officer if the patient is wary of any contact with the prison services. The *type of intervention* is usually informative and directive.

Of our therapies eight (12%) were more or less confined to this level. These patients could not be motivated to cooperate therapeutically, in the narrower sense; in a way they did not have the emotional reserves to enter into therapy.

Although this support is strictly speaking pretherapeutic, it is important and often very helpful. We mention this level, too, because it also occasionally crops up with other patients. Help of this kind can be important at the outset of therapy - for example, as a way of awakening a patient's trust in the therapist's solidarity and willingness to help; it can pave the way to future therapy. The therapist must be prepared not only to recognize the importance of these problems but also show active willingness to help solve them.

4.4.2.2 Help in Coping with Current Crises

This *therapeutic task* involves dealing with and overcoming current and acute crises and conflicts such as suicidal crises, an impending or de facto separation from a partner, major conflicts with parents, etc. The *type of intervention* is crisis intervention. The therapeutic focus is on the acute crisis, the approach is mainly ego-supportive. This support can be limited to help in coping with difficulties in the patient's social life, or can place greater emphasis on attempting to develop coping strategies for these crises. In 10 cases (14%) therapy was limited to this kind of crisis intervention; it was not possible to deal with more extensive problems. As on the first level, the focus was on current needs and requirements. Concentrating on crisis intervention can help these patients, and is sometimes all that is required, as the sexual symptom is often a "crisis coping strategy" and recedes once ongoing crises have been overcome.

Case 1 (see p. 32 for previous history)

Tormented by guilt feelings about his offence (sexual acts with his adopted daughters), this patient was still deeply depressed and full of self-reproach and shame at the start of therapy. He was still suffering from the effects of an attempted suicide 1½ years earlier (tracheostoma, respiratory and speech problems). His prison sentence (postponed on medical grounds) hung over him like the sword of Damocles and constantly revived his wish to kill himself. He was offered support immediately. In the 12 sessions therapy focussed on two tasks: on the first level (help in coping with social circumstances) we first succeeded with a petition to absolve the patient from his prison sentence. This was a great relief to the patient, not only because the external danger had been removed but also because the therapist's (successful) efforts on his behalf helped him to see his offence not only in a moral light but also as an expression of his plight at the time of the crisis. In the second phase (crisis intervention) the crisis was reconstructed and was easier to understand (regressive withdrawal to a childlike position in relation to his wife whom he felt was superior, overdemanding and contemptuous about his virility). This enabled him to understand the crisis as part of his past which he had got over and gave him the freedom to turn his attention to his future prospects. Once he had overcome the suicidal crisis, the patient decided to terminate therapy.

In a follow-up session about 1 year later the patient reported that he was getting on well, had regained a firm footing in his job and was about to remarry. Deviant desires had not reoccurred; he considered them only to be a part of the critical developments during his first marriage which he had in the meantime overcome.

In summary, therapy dealt solely with his current situation and depressive decompensation. The underlying problem was basically left untouched. Although therapy was restricted to crisis intervention, it appears to have been sufficient to restabilize the patient.

Here, as with the first level, it is clear that aspects of crisis intervention are involved in many therapies and, depending on what is required, frequently form a component of therapeutic work on the different levels.

4.4.2.3 Focus on Current Behaviour and Feelings

Neurotic symptoms, anxieties, inhibitions and conflicts manifested in definable situations as concrete behaviour form the subject and *focus* of therapy. *Intervention* aims at structuring the situation. In behaviourist terms this is the *level of the horizontal approach,* as described by Grawe and Dziewas (1977). The aim is to differentiate the patient's experience and perception of his behaviour patterns and the circumstances invoking them (classical horizontal behaviour analysis), and to provide him with practical coping strategies in critical situations when he usually resorts to destructive forms of behaviour and develops typical perverse or nonperverse symptoms. Instructions on how to behave and client-centred techniques are used to encourage differentiated self-perception. This approach can help the patient to identify and start working on his anxieties and deficits. The therapeutic goal is not just to modify behaviour in specific situations, but to practise dealing with critical situations and thereby acquire competence to help him cope outside therapy. Of our therapies 38 (55%) concentrated on this level.

It is vitally important not to resort automatically to behaviour therapy techniques for symptom control or behaviour modification such as are found in preplanned programmes, but rather to use these techniques selectively within the framework of an evolving therapeutic gestalt. This presupposes an analysis of the patient-therapist relationship and the psychodynamic implications of these techniques. If, as often happens, the patient repeatedly thwarts the therapist's attempts to structure his approach, it is essential to reassess the patient's resistance and anxieties and perhaps even revise the therapeutic procedure. We shall now discuss the various aspects which can be tackled by means of elements from behaviour therapy: the perverse symptom, the patient's partner relationship, and problematic forms of social behaviour.

The Perverse Symptom as the Focus of Therapy

Even though we attribute key significance to a psychodynamic understanding of the perverse symptom when working towards a gestalt, this does not necessarily mean that the symptom is chronologically the first focus or significant enough to be the central focus in therapy. The fact that the perverse symptom is, as a rule, the reason why a patient seeks therapy may tempt one to give the symptom the highest priority. This temptation should however be resisted. A therapist should carefully consider, particularly from the psychodynamic angle, when and even whether the perverse symptom should be discussed at all and in which stage of the therapy, and which interventions and techniques are appropriate.

Case 4 (see page 41 for previous history)

After we had written an expertise on this patient, he was unexpectedly released from prison. His wife had ceased to care about him and was considering leaving him. A few days after being released the patient was admitted as an inpatient to a psychiatric clinic after a suicide attempt. This happened after a bitter argument with his wife. The threat of losing his home filled him with panic, all the more so since he had also lost his job. After a few inpatient *crisis intervention sessions* treatment was continued on an outpatient basis. The next 10 sessions with a male therapist were dominated by his hopelessness and self-reproach. The patient accused himself of having prejudiced not only his own, but also his wife's existence and destroyed their mutual happiness. He no longer had any self-respect and felt physically ill: he had tried drinking alcohol to "treat" his heart and stomach complaints as well as his separation anxieties, but this only caused further tension. He was so preoccupied with his current problems that the sexual offences he felt very ashamed of could not be discussed, as the confrontation would have dramatically amplified the crisis. As the therapist considered it essential to stabilize the patient's personal situation, and the patient's wife now felt less certain about the separation, he suggested *couple therapy* which both accepted. Therapy with this couple lasted 1½ years (52 sessions). The separation problem was soon solved; the couple decided to stay together. The wife at first participated half-heartedly and saw herself as a kind of co-therapist, but soon found that she herself benefitted. Her husband's attempts to bully and restrict her, her opposition and her ensuing submission became the main focus of therapy. She was encouraged in her wish to create a life of her own independently of her husband. At the time she was catching up on her secondary school diploma and planned to go to university. The patient was able to accept this after realizing that his own insecurity and fear of being abandoned lay behind his need to dominate and control her and that precisely this lack of trust had led to the estrangement between the two partners. The relationship became more trusting and reciprocal; the patient seemed distinctly more open and spontaneous. He also succeeded in finding employment again. The sexual symptoms were excluded until the very end of therapy. The central problem underlying his perverse symptom became clear to him during couple therapy: adaptation to a different culture, fear of women who he regarded as superior, and impulses to take revenge on them, plus a deep-rooted doubt in his masculinity inherited from childhood. The perverse symptoms did not reappear during therapy.

In the 3-year follow-up period the patient was suspected once of voyeurism. He dismissed this suspicion, seemed well-balanced and pleased with his marriage and career.

To summarize, in this therapy the patient's resistance to discussing the symptom was respected. Confronting the patient's impaired self-esteem with the symptom of which he was so ashamed would have been too much for him and would probably have deepened his depressive crisis again. Bringing in his wife and working through the partnership problems gave him support and self-confidence. In this increasingly relaxed situation it was possible to focus on the male identity anxieties dating from childhood, which had been reactivated during the process of integrating into a new culture. The improved mutual understanding gave the marriage a new basis. It was still uncertain whether the perversion, being an unhealed wound, would not erupt again in a crisis.

When deciding whether behaviour therapy techniques should be used to control symptoms, it is important to closely analyse the kind of symptoms and their roots in personality structure. *Three aspects of the symptom* are of particular interest here: first, the kind of struggle between the personality and the symptom, e.g. the kind of *inner coping*, second, the *acuteness or intensity* of the perverse symptom and, finally, the degree of the patient's *dependency on the perverse symptom.*

As far as the kinds of inner coping are concerned, we refer the reader to Sect. 3.2.1.2 in which we described a continuum between the ego-syntonic and ego-dystonic poles. The kind of coping involved has a direct influence on the chances for therapeutic access.

Obviously, an emphasis on *ego-syntonic coping* in a patient means he will be more or less unwilling to cooperate for instance in exercises to aid symptom control, even if he verbally and emphatically asserts the opposite when worried by a pending trial. This soon becomes obvious in unambiguous ego-syntonic coping, which was seldom found and then usually in convinced pedophiles. More irritating for the therapist are those patients whose positive attitude towards their symptom is less open and frank, but more secretive and ambiguous (for example some exhibitionists; see Case 8, p. 107). One often only becomes aware of this later when, for example, the patient repeatedly forgets appointments, although superficially he seems willing to cooperate.

At the other end of the scale, *ego-dystonic or ego-alien coping* presents the therapist with different problems. The desire to get rid of the symptom is in this case paramount and often the only reason for starting therapy. These patients reject their symptom and respond to it with disgust, guilt feelings and anxieties of varying intensity. They cannot reconcile it with their self-image; many feel at first that talking about their problem does not provide relief; on the contrary it is humiliating and shameful and something which they try to avoid or consciously subject themselves to - as it were as "deserved punishment". A therapist who fails to notice this, sticks to his therapy plan and, for example, persists in carrying out his analysis of the patient's behaviour, can help intensify the patient's already negative view of himself and allow him to get entangled even further in feelings of depression and self-hatred. In these cases the therapist should aim at helping the patient to talk more freely about his symptom, without insisting on it.

Apart from the kind of symptom coping, *the acuteness or intensity of the perverse symptom* is another important factor in deciding whether symptom control methods are appropriate. Here, too, there is a wide range of possibilities. At the one end we had patients whose deviant act in an acute psychic crisis was *a unique and isolated event*. Some patients experienced deviant desires or impulsive outbursts more or less infrequently and sporadically and were sometimes quite free of them during therapy; in others sexual activity was frequently associated and linked with perverse desires and phantasies. Finally, at the other extreme the patients' symptoms became increasingly severe; they felt a compulsive desire which came in waves; they felt they could not resist these impulses, but were driven and overwhelmed by them.

A third, extremely important aspect in working out a therapeutic concept is *the patient's dependency on the perverse symptom*, i.e. the degree to which a patient is dependent on the symptom for his psychic equilibrium. There are patients who, without necessarily being aware it, doggedly resist relinquishing their symptom even though they regard it as a burden on a more cognitive level. Patients' thoughts of "losing" their symptom in therapy are coupled with anxieties about forfeiting an important way of finding new courage in critical situations; the perverse enactment gives them a sense of awareness and a vitality which are otherwise sealed off and cannot be experienced. These anxieties, which are at first more or less hidden, affect many patients, but are usually concealed behind the equally prevalent desire on another level to overcome the humiliating symptom.

These three aspects of the symptom and its roots in personality structure which have to be analysed represent only one side of the coin. One also has to consider the *type and quality of the patient-therapist relationship* when deciding whether behaviour therapy techniques focussing on the sexual symptom are appropriate. This means deciding whether the therapeutic relationship is already robust enough to allow the patient to overcome his inner barriers and inhibitions and talk about the humiliating symptom without fear of losing the therapist's esteem. Does the patient over-idealize the therapist, delegate responsibility for the symptom onto the therapist, and project magic powers of symptom removal onto him? What might be the possible effects of behaviour therapy methods on the patient-therapist relationship?

These considerations make it quite clear that one cannot lay down rigid or universal rules and regulations for developing a therapeutic gestalt and deciding in favour of or against behaviour therapy for treating the symptom. Structuring therapy is a far too individual process, is far too dependent on the patient's individual problem and on the exigencies of a specific therapeutic situation. As regards *selecting behaviourist methods,* in our view purely *aversive techniques and methods* and measuring techniques (such as phallometry) are for psychodynamic reasons clearly unsuitable. They are in any case only accepted, and indeed frequently requested, by patients who have an extremely negative attitude toward their symptom combined with deep self-hatred and the impulse to punish themselves. Using aversive techniques would mean taking the same negative stance and reinforcing it, helping act out the punishment impulses, taking over the role of the immature superego and merging the role of therapist with that of a penal institution. This would frustrate from the very start any hope of psychotherapeutic work on the problems linked to the symptom.

Accordingly, we confined ourselves to methods of *self-control* (horizontal behaviour analysis, base line, thought stopping, stimulus control). These methods are only useful if the symptom is active during therapy, the patient's way of coping is not too close to the ego-syntonic pole and he no longer feels (quite as) dependent on the symptom.

From the psychodynamic angle the decision to use symptom-control techniques means adopting at first the patient's negative attitude towards his symptom, in part isolating and objectifying the symptom, appealing to the patient's self-control, his willingness to make an effort and his responsibility for himself as well as temporarily dispensing with interpretation. This approach, combined with the patient's increasingly differentiated perception of the inward and outward causes of the symptom can gradually deprive the symptom of its alien character. Experiencing the perverse desires and impulses, inner tension, anxieties, feelings of anger, distress, inner void etc. encourages a more accepting view of the symptom. This also gives the patient a new insight into his symptom and a way of understanding it, not along moral lines, but as an expression of his problem. This method is often helpful when the symptom becomes more severe. The growing certainty of being able to control impulses, of being reinstated as one's own master, can decisively help to raise the patient's self-esteem.

Restricting therapy to the level of horizontal behaviour analysis using self-control methods can be especially productive. This holds particularly for patients who have little access to their own emotions hidden in the symptom, who are very afraid of confronting themselves with their own problems and "weaknesses" and resist any introspection. Instead, these patients cling to their achievements and are proud of their strengths and autonomy. Methods for improving self-control give them the feeling that they can actively do something about their symptom (see Case 10, p. 111; 13, p. 95; 17, p. 91).

Case 8 (see p. 49 for previous history)

This patient, who had already had 2 years of psychoanalytic treatment with no effect on his symptoms, came to therapy on his own initiative as he had noticed that after separating from his wife he was no longer able to control his exhibitionist desires, which were increasing and taking on a life of their own. As he had a long way to travel, sessions took place at large intervals (fortnightly to monthly) over a 1-year period, including one therapy block of several days. The patient was worried that he no longer had a grip on his exhibitionism and that he was in danger of being overwhelmed by the increasingly frequent urge to expose himself - a very difficult situation for a distinctly intellectual and self-controlled person. He was not interested in discovering the inner roots of his symptom, but wanted to learn how to deal with exhibiting in such a way as not to jeopardize himself and his career. The (female) therapist sensed the immense vulnerability he was trying to cover up. He rebuffed cautious attempts at discussing the feelings hidden behind his intellectual, factual façade (e.g. his reactions to his wife leaving him). Therapy was defined by the patient from the very beginning as a kind of workshop.

The method chosen for therapy was symptom control as the patient's initial motivation was his fear of no longer being able to control the symptom. He became aware that he could steer therapy himself and that he was not dependent on the therapist. In the intervals between sessions he followed suggestions and programmes eagerly and even enlarged on them. As symptom control grew, his self-esteem gradually recovered.

The patient's zealous cooperation caused the therapist to encourage him not to fight too hard against his symptom. For the patient, who had himself never seriously questioned his exhibitionism, this was unexpected confirmation which further stabilized him.

Follow-up after 3½ years showed that the patient had maintained the improvement achieved during therapy. He was still exposing himself, although seldom, in a "harmless" ritual of his own choice. All in all, he seemed more open, had a steady girlfriend again and was less obsessed by work and being a success.

To summarize, this patient's problem was less the symptom itself than his inability to control his perverse impulses on his own. This narcissistic insult was ultimately the driving force behind treatment. The level of approach - behaviour therapy techniques for coping practically with the ego-syntonic symptom - coincided with the patient's wishes; he continued nonetheless to hide behind his intellectualization of the problem.

To what extent restriction to the horizontal symptom level is useful or adequate can only be assessed on a case-by-case basis. Horizontal behaviour analysis and symptom control are helpful as two elements in a growing therapeutic gestalt as this approach can be the first, preparatory step in enabling the patient to gain a broader understanding of the symptomatic character of his perverse behaviour.

Behaviour Therapy for Couples

Our reason for discussing the problems of a behaviour therapy approach taking the perverse symptom as an example is that the approach is of major importance both in the literature and in therapeutic practice. The same applies equally when other matters troubling the patient, such as partnership problems or social contacts, are taken as the focus of therapy.

In terms of frequency, couple therapy plays a major role in our therapies. A patient's basic problem, such as relating to others, doubting his maleness and dealing with aggressive feelings, as well as his most important coping strategies, can be easily recognized in the way he behaves towards his spouse and are experienced vividly by both partners; in fact, many patients find it easier to understand them in this context than as part of the perverse symptom. Couple therapy is particularly advisable when the patient's partner also suffers from the relationship pattern, her part in it is perceptible and she feels she herself could benefit from therapy.

Using the level of the couple's actual, current behaviour and feelings, communicative interaction and partner sexuality offer a starting point for therapy. When *focussing on partner interaction* , the place to start is their practical interaction, hindered by strategies such as withdrawal, excessive harmony, delegation of responsibility, control, submission, etc. One can make use of *communication exercises* if the patients (and the therapist) are amenable to them. This may apply particularly when the partners find it difficult to reach their own emotions. Here, too, the therapist has to go beyond the immediate behaviour level to understand them. In some cases one can succeed in identifying and formulating the couple's specific wishes and anxieties and help them to develop a new relationship plan.

The modifications of the Masters-Johnson therapy described by Arentewicz and Schmidt (1983) proved extremely helpful when *partner sexuality* was the focus of therapy. Most of the partnerships were unerotic; sexual contact was avoided; this may be superficially a relief, but is usually combined with dissatisfaction and tension. In this field, too, a behaviourist approach helps to give the therapist a deeper insight into the patient's difficulties.

Case 14 (see p. 63 for previous history)

This patient had been previously convicted for indecent exposure to women; a new trial was pending. He experienced his symptom as something shameful and alien which threatened his respectable, success-oriented world. He was afraid his symptom would destroy his whole existence which he had so far held together by strictly obeying conventions.

We decided to involve his wife in treatment and start couple therapy for the following reasons: the patient's symptom functioned as a counterbalance to the life to which he had reconciled himself, in which instinctual drives and intimacy were taboo. Even marriage, in which the partners were still estranged, failed to satisfy his longing for intimacy and acceptance as a man. Sexuality played practically no role at all. Couple therapy was started with the aim of integrating a less pathological and distorted form of sexuality into the relationship and helping the partners to draw closer to one another. Sexuality was understood as a vehicle and mode of expression for the couple's basic desires and anxieties.

Over a 2-year period 55 sessions were held with a male and female therapist. The wife was spontaneously cooperative and she quickly understood her own problems (skin disease, alcohol) as the expression of joint difficulties. While the partners practised a cautious physical approach in exercises adapted from Masters and Johnson, the desires and anxieties involved in the rapprochement were discussed. Both partners avoided giving up their passivity and moving toward one another. One could see how the patient had mixed up sexuality with aggression and was constantly afraid of offending his wife by touching her. Gradually both learnt to perceive their own psychic and physical reactions more precisely and to start a dialogue. In doing so, they partially succeeded in coping with disagreements with less fear and greater openness. Although both still felt that sexuality played a subordinate role, the growing emotional intimacy enriched the relationship. The patient's wish to expose himself faded more and more into the background.

No deviant acts had occurred again 2 years after completing therapy. The relationship had stabilized; both had come out of their social isolation by joining a charity organization.

To summarize, treatment succeeded in showing the couple their fears and longings hidden in the symptom and in dealing with them. This led to mutual relief and made the symptom, which we interpreted as an expression of a *disturbance in the relationship,* superfluous.

Problematic Forms of Social Behaviour

On the behavioural level, one can also focus on the problems a patient has in social interaction: coping with life, a depressive outlook, isolation, self-destructive tendencies, fixation on success, a dreary and monotonous daily routine, etc. Using the patient's actual behaviour and feelings, the therapist intervenes, aiming at: internalizing ways of asserting oneself, coping with conflicts, making contact and shaping a relationship; reducing fears of failure and contact; differentiating and correcting the patient's perception and idea of himself. The relationship to the therapist can be an important testing ground for these processes. We made use of various methods to *improve self-confidence and contact* and to *reduce anxiety,* which we adapted individually to each patient and his problem, and also client-centred methods for *differentiating perception of emotions* . Here, too, the therapist has to grasp the underlying conflicts behind the more superficial anxieties, behaviour deficits and cognitive structures to avoid the risk of superficial training. By using specific behaviours and immediate experience, it often proves possible to make the patient aware of deeper anxieties and help him question his set ideas on himself and his world.

Case 12 (see p. 60 for previous history)

As the patient lived far away he was admitted to an open psychiatric ward for 6 weeks. Apart from the 27 day sessions with a male therapist, he took part in social and therapeutic activities on the ward. After being discharged, support sessions took place every month over a period of 1 ¼ years.

The patient had broken off psychoanalytic treatment in his home town and was highly ambivalent about beginning therapy again. He was cool, monosyllabic, overly cautious, resigned and guarded. The therapist sensed his high vulnerability and inner loneliness and tried carefully to make contact and gain his trust. The therapeutic situation was at first comparable with an empathic father supporting his shy and reserved son.

The main problem soon became clear: the symptom was the patient's only way of filling his colourless inner world with life and giving himself a sense of worth by caring for the boys he courted. Despite the extreme, desperately felt urgency of his pedophile desires, it did not seem advisable to focus on the perverse symptom. The patient wavered constantly between a desire for the "magic" removal of the symptom and, at the same time, a deep fear of losing his only opportunity for making contact and taking part in social life. His participation in life on the ward forced him to adapt and make (superficial) contacts. A plan was worked out with the patient to help him overcome his inhibitions step by step. The therapist gave him the task of attending events, talking to people and making appointments. The patient's experiences, his fears of rejection and his inferiority feelings were discussed in sessions and he began to be aware of his (suppressed) desire to be accepted and protected. He was gradually able to take a more relaxed stance toward the therapist, even though he repeatedly withdrew. When he successfully fulfilled the agreed "tasks", he felt a little better and more secure. It was then possible to look at his fears of having to prove his virility to women while cautiously approaching the symptom and starting a discussion on his physical aversions to and phantasies about women.

At follow-up 2 years after completing therapy, the patient reported that he had at first sporadically sought contact to young boys, but not as compulsively; this need had, however, faded into the background since he had started a relationship with a woman for the first time. He was capable of coping with greater demands in his new job and had a distinctly more realistic view on life.

To summarize, treatment in this case was a corrective emotional experience: the patient was offered help in dealing with his anxiety-ridden reality on a behavioural level. The therapist became a well-wishing "father" who accepted the patient with his weakness and was trusted. Treatment was *ego-supportive* and did not deal with the aggressive side of his personality. The patient was able to see in the therapist an aspect of positive and loving masculinity and to identify with him.

Finally, we should again like to emphasize the following point: although we have discussed various aspects of the symptom and the behaviour therapy methods chosen, they should not be mistaken for pieces in a mosaic as in the multi-dimensional approach we criticized. At least ideally, making use of any specific technique should stem from the broadest possible understanding of the patient and his psychodynamic situation – in the interest of a carefully considered and individually tailored therapeutic approach. Therapy should not be restricted to the level of current behaviour and feelings just because the therapist lacks insight. Therapy consisting only of a string of techniques would become a haphazard game with an uncertain outcome. Our results also provide arguments against a multi-dimensional approach by showing that successful therapies in fact focussed on only one or very few areas. Although the therapies varied greatly, the procedure within any given therapy was relatively uniform: in most therapies (58%) only one main focus was chosen, in some (38%) two, but almost never more. This seems to demonstrate the heuristic value of analysing the meaning of the symptom. A simple stringing together of techniques is usually a sign of therapeutic disorientation which, in the worst cases, leads to polypragmatic activity for its own sake which is paramount to failure.

4.4.2.4 *Identifying Emotional Contexts, Overall Behaviour Patterns and Functional Connections*

We have already pointed out several times that behaviour therapy methods may provide a useful entry to a broader understanding of the patient's problems. The attempt to understand the symptom and use this as the basis and orientation for therapeutic procedure is not just relevant at the start of therapy, but continues to be a crucial factor in therapeutic planning during the entire therapy. Ideally the ongoing therapeutic procedure and a deepening understanding of the symptom should augment one another. Very often further facets of the meaning of the symptom emerge during therapy, especially if one succeeds in extending the range of the therapy. In some cases we were able to get beyond the more superficial emotions, such as fears of failure and social insecurity, etc., and discovered more deep-seated anxieties about relationships and basic existential fears. In 13 of our therapies (19%)[5] we managed to probe beyond merely understanding and gaining control over specific symptoms and helped the patient to understand the context. In these cases we could, for instance, show that the perverse symptom highlights a problem which is also manifested in other ways in social anxiety, phantasies and difficulties in relationships. We were then able to trace how the patient's problem evolved from his developmental and social history. The *style of intervention* we chose was interpretative and confronting.

In behaviourist terminology the fourth level extends the horizontal to include the vertical approach, as described by Grawe and Dziewas (1977).

Case 10 (see p. 57 for previous history)

Individual therapy, complemented by couple therapy, lasted 68 sessions over a 2½-year period.

Initially the patient was passive and helpless; he seemed to have handed over the entire responsiblity for himself to the therapist. The patient felt utterly worthless and insignificant. He had an extremely guilty conscience because of his compulsive, perverse desires (voyeurism).

In the first phase the therapist decided to support the patient on the *level of current behaviour and feelings* by giving him instructions. This seemed the best approach for several reasons: interpretation and confrontation would have tended to confirm the patient's unstable, negative self-image rather than enable him to discover new perspectives. His subordination to and idealization of the therapist suggested an active approach was called for, without supporting his passivity. Appealing to the patient's sense of responsibility for himself activated him, and the discovery that he could influence and control his behaviour gave him self-confidence. As he was deeply ashamed of the perverse symptom and had an extremely negative attitude towards it, his social awkwardness was chosen as the first main focus. The more he overcame his insecurity and inhibitions, the more his perverse desires receded. In the *second phase,* attention turned to *analysing the symptom and its meaning.* The patient began to understand that he reversed his impotence in the perversion by observing sleeping, defenceless women and in doing so sensed a power and superiority he was otherwise unable to experience. Supported by his relationship to the therapist, he began resisting his wife's watchful guard over him. He realized

---

[5] The therapy figures quoted for the four levels add up to n = 69 and not n = 86, as 17 therapies could not be clearly assigned to any of the four levels.

that the relationship to his wife was as constrictive as that to his mother earlier. His perverse desires vanished in this phase, which lasted about 1 year. However, the patient's new self-confidence provoked fierce reactions in his wife: the marriage was jeopardized by their quarrelling. His wife was brought into the *third phase of therapy*. *Couple therapy* focussed on how both of them restricted and clung to one another. His wife began to understand that her own dependency made her sneer at her husband. As their mutual understanding increased, they were able to accept each other better. Although sexuality was not a focus in the therapy, the patient's erection dysfunction vanished and his wife had an orgasm for the first time.

Towards the end of therapy, the patient's acting out became problematic: he endangered himself by taking high risks, driving without a licence and disregarding traffic regulations. In the *final phase of therapy* the *relationship to the therapist* was the main theme. The patient tried to cope with his fear of separation by demonstrating to the therapist how heavily dependent he still was on him and that he wanted to delegate responsibility for himself onto the therapist. The latter cautiously rejected this delegation; in this situation the aggressive aspects behind the idealization emerged quite distinctly.

After therapy the application to remit his prison sentence was approved and he was pardoned. The patient was able to maintain his stability in the 2½-year follow-up period.

To summarize, by identifying with the therapist (the longed-for, idealized father), the patient gained acceptance and support in the conflict with his wife and other disputes. The security the therapist gave him helped him try out new experiences which contributed to his self-esteem. Couple therapy restored the equilibrium of the marriage which had been upset by the patient's stabilization. Finally, in the last phase of treatment his masochistic acting out was understood as an expression of separation anxieties and the main problem - the desire for dependency - was rejected in the transference relationship without causing any new traumatization.

Although we listed our four levels of approach and analysed statistically how frequently we used them, the figures themselves have little relevance. Essentially, they are a retrospective illustration of our therapeutic work in this project. The preponderance of the third level shows that this research project was originally given a behaviourist slant and that, besides client-centred therapy, the therapists were trained in behaviour therapy. As the project developed and the emphasis shifted to a psychodynamic approach, the fourth level was used more often. When we state that therapy on the fourth level only took place with one fifth of patients, this does not mean that an interpretative procedure was not feasible for the other four fifths. The numerical ratios do not present a realistic picture of therapeutic possiblities. This does not, however, detract from the validity of all four levels which show in distilled form the possibilities and limits of therapy for these patients.

It might be tempting to see a hierarchy in the four levels - which would fit in with an ideal concept of therapy and psychological health. However, an ideal concept of this kind is of little help in practical therapeutic work. It is an illusion to suppose the higher the level the better the therapy, the broader the level of access the more successful and stable the outcome. Our results and experience demonstrate impressively that the choice of level is not entirely a decision made by the therapist. It is first and foremost the patient and his problem which determine the level of therapy. The more serious the patient's pathology, and the less his willingness to undergo therapy, the more constructive it is to choose a lower level of approach as this offers the best chance of helping him.

The choice of level therefore depends on various exigencies, circumstances and requirements: the patient's pathology, his capacity for insight, the kind of patient-therapist relationship, the patient's anxiety and his willingness to question himself but also his current social situation and distress. The choice of level is by no means an initiative taken by the therapist. Which level of therapeutic approach is suitable for any specific combination of patient-therapist only starts emerging as the therapeutic gestalt develops. Consequently, the point is not to strive for the highest level, but instead to find out what can be usefully done under the given circumstances.

Moreover, the levels described are not rigid categories, but rather thematic and methodical focal points between which one can switch at any stage in therapy.

We should like to make one final point. Whether the complex process in which the therapeutic gestalt evolves is successful or not, whether the therapist grasps the context needed to understand the patient, depends essentially on the therapist's personality. This is an obvious point to make, but deserves particular mention in this context. Carrying out therapy with these patients, whose symptoms infringe on the therapist's emotional life and value systems, makes high demands on her/his powers of reflection and flexibility in an especially demanding situation where she/he too is under surveillance (see Sect. 4.2.). Patients with sexually deviant symptoms confront the therapist with the cracks in her/his own autonomy and normative convictions; this can trigger a great deal of fear and activate the therapists' defence mechanisms which can prevent therapy progressing.

"Flooding" the patient with emotional warmth, which is often combined with unrealistic rescue phantasies or an allegedly flexible therapy plan, and typically switches constantly between new techniques, is nothing more than an attempt to control fears which the patient has activated in the therapist. This illustrates the immense importance of *continual supervison* for the therapists of such patients. Supervision should be oriented psychodynamically, irrespective of the therapist's approach and take account of the multilateral pressure exerted on the therapist by the patient's demands, by society and law enforcement and her/his own normative attitudes. Empathic understanding - the prerequisite for a constructive patient-therapist relationship - can only develop if the therapist tries to face and deal with her/his own anxieties and defence mechanisms.

4.5 Results of Therapy

4.5.1 Preamble

We do not intend to enter into an endless discussion reviewing the almost overwhelming flood of literature on research into therapy outcome. This discussion will never reach a conclusion because the problem of measurability of therapy outcome, no matter how important it may be, cannot really be solved finally and completely. The reason for this lies in the (partial) incongruence between the measured factors and the criteria of measurement; the changes which make up the therapeutic process - potentially *qualitative* changes - can only be measured very approximately in terms of *quantity*. As a result, evaluation of outcome is already influenced to a large extent by the criteria selected (Cartwright and Roth 1957; Luborsky 1962; Strupp and Luborsky 1962; Mintz 1972). The assessment of the success of a therapy will vary greatly depending on the methods used, whether only the superficial symptom modifications or, additionally, modifications in personality are measured. It also depends on which personality modifications are considered particularly significant and are picked out because they fit in with a particular interpretation of the problem and the aim of therapy. The selection made depends in turn on the therapeutic team's focus of interest: are they concerned more about the patient's subjective satisfaction, the stability of changes or, especially in therapy for delinquents, about society's interests?

The methodological incongruence in experimental therapy designs is obvious when a patient sample, whose symptoms manifest a homogenous problem, is put through a comparable or more or less standardized therapy programme. Even if this incongruence can be reduced to an acceptable level experimentally in these programmes, this will not succeed nearly as well in clinical research of therapeutic processes. However, our patient group was nonhomogenous in many respects:

- Differences in deviant symptoms in both type and intensity varying between the extremes of increasing severity and a single lapse in a crisis situation
- Differences in personality structure ranging from relatively stable and slightly disturbed personalities to patients with serious borderline pathologies
- Differences in therapeutic procedure ranging from short therapies lasting a few hours which focussed on help in coping with everyday life or crisis interventions to year-long therapies in which the problem, reflected in the therapist-patient relationship, was interpreted and worked through.

Uniform rating criteria for therapy outcome control can therefore only provide a very incomplete picture of the therapeutic process and modifications which can be measured at the close of therapy.

This sceptical preamble is not, however, meant as a plea for dispensing with an assessment of the outcome of therapy altogether, but merely emphasizes the limitations of the methodological approach.

When rating therapy success, especially therapy for sex offenders, two groups of criteria are involved: *internal* and *external criteria*. Internal criteria include the two categories *differential modification criteria* and *overall evaluation of therapy outcome*; external criteria are *relapse quota* and *psychophysiological measurements*.

Internal Therapy Criteria

Differential Modification Criteria. In differential measurement of change single aspects of a patient's personality are isolated - for example, the acuteness and intensity of specific symptoms, certain personality areas, etc. - and recorded separately. Values are calculated at the close of therapy and at follow-up and compared with pretherapy values. This method of measuring outcome has the advantage of greater transparency and therefore makes the therapy results easier to verify. The disadvantage is that the patient's personality is, as it were, divided up into separate, seemingly disconnected aspects - a kind of atomization which can obscure insight into the overall context. Moreover, the meaning of the modifications in each separate aspect can vary from patient to patient. Concluding that "the deviant symptom does not reappear" at the end of therapy, for example, says nothing about therapy success with patients whose deviant act occurred only once or sporadically as a way of coping with crises and who otherwise have no deviant desires. Rating a tendency to depression at the end of therapy is irrelevant for assessing outcome if a pronounced defence against depression is one of the patient's main problems. Good job and social integration say nothing about the quality of therapy for patients who were in any case assessed positively and considered stable.

Overall Evaluation of Therapy Outcome. The disadvantage of a lack of transparency in method when giving an overall assessment of therapy cannot be remedied even if one names the criteria on which evaluation is based. The advantage, however, is that therapeutic effects are related to the patient's individual problem and that one can avoid artificial subdivision into seemingly more precise and manageable component parts. In order to reduce subjectivity in such evaluations, we recommend that independent investigators, and not the therapists or the patients, assess the overall effect of therapy.

External Criteria

Relapse Rates. Although it is useful and necessary to include relapses in the evaluation of therapy outcome and thereby retain a perspective on the real situation and the social consequences, it is important to understand that this is a criterion alien to therapy. Seen critically, the absence of a relapse is by no means a criterion of success, nor is a relapse proof of no success - ignoring for a moment the problems with the figures for unrecorded cases and the pure chance of an offence being discovered or prosecuted. If relapse rate is taken as the only or central criterion of success it is clear that the researcher's interests coincide with those of society's penal institutions. "If one uses this form of success evaluation one undoubtedly runs the risk ... of confusing the criteria of therapy with the principles of disciplinarian thinking whose objective is not to restore a healthy personality, but primarily to do away with an incriminating symptom" (Petri 1980, p. 209).

Psychophysiological measurements. Measuring the phallus to gauge patient arousability under experimentally defined deviant stimuli is a recurrent topic in the literature, especially for sex offenders. After all we have said about our diagnostic and therapeutic concept, there is little more we can do to explain why we consider this method completely inappropriate, for a number of reasons. Disregarding for a moment the methodological problems of how to obtain reliable results, this method is evidence of a fixation on the isolated symptom and represents a need to check on the patient which, in our view, can hardly be reconciled with a therapeutic approach. We do not wish to go into the implications of using these methods in prognosis, release from prison and so on, nor into their striking similarity with the so-called lie-detector.

4.5.2 Methods and Results

Despite the reservations already mentioned, we decided to use both types of internal criteria and to report on both the *differential modification criteria* and *overall evaluation of therapy outcome*; of the external criteria we selected the *relapse rate*.

As regards internal criteria, we had three *sources of evaluation*: the *patients'* own assessment of various factors, the evaluation made by the *therapists* and the assessment made by an independent *rater group* (the authors). To avoid subjective distortion, we did not use patient and therapist assessment as a criterion for overall evaluation. *Restriction to the rater group* seems to us the most sensible approach as their assessment is certainly the most valid.

In Sect. 3.1.2 we described in detail the methods which the rater group used. We should like to repeat: after thoroughly studying all the information available on a patient, the raters - at first independently of each other - used the category system which had been worked out to assess the diagnosis, the therapist-patient relationship and the therapeutic process and, finally, the situation at the end of therapy and at follow-up. In joint group discussions we arrived at a consensus on our assessment of each patient. The outcome is described in our results. There were limits to the independence of the rater group in as much as one or two authors frequently knew the patient being assessed from therapy, initial interviews or follow-up sessions.

There was one disadvantage in rater assessment: it took place at one specific moment during the course of the project. It is therefore quite likely that our perception of differences over time was blurred, particularly between the end of therapy and follow-up; the therapists' assessments certainly differentiate better between these two points in time. One effect one has to expect is that negative information at the time of follow-up interferes with retrospective assessment of change during therapy, and vice versa. This inaccuracy has to be accepted.

4.5.2.1 *Follow-ups*

Follow-up reports were available for 51 of 86 patients (59%). The time between the end of therapy and follow-up ranged from 6 months to 7 years, the mean being 2⅓ years ($\bar{x}=2.4$; $s=1.5$; median = 2.2 years; Table 10).

Table 10. Distribution of follow-up time

Period	n	%
½-1 year	10	20
1-2 years	17	33
2-3 years	7	13
3-4 years	12	24
More than 4 years	5	10
No follow-up	35	
Total	86	100

To test for biased selection in the follow-up sample we analysed the variables significantly related to therapy outcome to see if the sample was composed differently from the subsample for which we had no follow-up data. The overall assessment of therapies by the rater group was taken as an indicator of therapy success. Our analysis showed that the follow-up sample did not differ significantly from the sample without follow-up. The follow-up sample can be seen as representative for the entire group.

4.5.2.2 *Analysis of Control Group*

Patients on the waiting list were used as a control group. We are aware that this method does not provide us with an optimal check for our data. The waiting period before a patient starts therapy cannot be seen as a neutral, irrelevant phase (see also Baekeland and Lundwall, 1975; Luborsky et al. 1971). The prospects of getting help, patients' hopes and disappointments during the waiting

Table 11. Distribution of waiting period

Time	n	%
0-6 months	31	38
7-12 months	30	36
13-18 months	10	12
More than 18 months	11	14
No information	4	
Total	86	100

period can lead to an improvement or deterioration in the symptoms. The validity is also restricted by the immense differences in the length of the waiting period (Table 11).

On average, patients waited just under 9 months for therapy; standard deviation was s=7 months.

We decided nonetheless in favour of a control group because it is the only ethically acceptable method in clinical psychotherapy research.

The current acuteness and intensity of the deviant symptoms were evaluated at the initial interview and at the beginning and end of therapy (Tables 12, 13).[6]

A comparison of the groups showed no significant differences in the distribution of the symptoms prior to therapy. As regards distribution of individual symptom changes, there was no indication of any significant deterioration or improvement (sign test). With all due caution, we consider this to be some indication of the validity of our therapy results.

Table 12a. Acuteness of deviant desires (therapist assessment)

Frequency of desires	Initial interview (n=86)		Therapy start (n=86)	
	n	%	n	%
No desires	10	13	12	17
Up to once per month	17	21	12	17
Up to several a week	36	45	32	45
More often	17	21	15	21
Not assessable	6		15	
Total	86	100	86	100

Table 12b. Acuteness of deviant desires (therapist assessment)

Frequency of desires	Therapy end (n=86)		Follow-up (n=51)	
	n	%	n	%
No desires	28	37	20	42
Up to once per month	21	28	13	27
Up to several a week	22	29	13	27
More often	5	6	2	4
Not assessable	10		3	
Total	86	100	51	100

[6] This is based on therapist assessment since separate rater assessment for initial interviews and start of therapy is not available and, in retrospect, was not feasible.

Table 13a. Acuteness of deviant behaviour (therapist assessment)

Frequency of behaviour	Initial interview (n=86)		Therapy start (n=86)	
	n	%	n	%
Not acute	15	20	22	33
Up to once per month	33	45	23	34
Up to several a week	23	31	16	24
More often	3	4	6	9
Not assessable	12		19	
Total	86	100	86	100

Table 13b. Acuteness of deviant behaviour (therapist assessment)

Frequency of behaviour	Therapy end (n=86)		Follow-up (n=51)	
	n	%	n	%
Not acute	45	60	29	59
Up to once per month	18	24	12	25
Up to several a week	11	15	7	14
More often	1	1	1	2
Not assessable	11		2	
Total	86	100	51	100

4.5.2.3 Differential Measurement of Changes

In spite of all the objections and limitations to the validity of the data we isolated and assessed the following aspects: the *acuteness of the deviant symptoms, social and occupational integration,* subjective *sexual satisfaction* and *neurotic symptom formation,* such as alcoholism, tendency to depression and psychosomatic symptoms. On the evidence of the material we had, no major changes to the test values had occurred either at the close of therapy or at follow-up.

Change in Deviant Symptoms

Tables 14 and 15 point to the following conclusions: the deviant symptom was considered still highly acute in one third of the patients; no essential change was observed in comparison with their initial situation. An improvement was seen in two thirds of the patients. One third was free of symptoms at the end of therapy. There are noticeable differences within the improved group. The category "distinctly improved" means that although deviant desires occasionally emerge they can be controlled. Combining this group with the symptom-free group, one can say that therapy was clearly successful, in terms of the symptom, for over half the patients. A comparison between the end of therapy and follow-up shows that the changes were stable.

In view of the differences among the patient groups, a comparison with other studies is hardly possible. There are a few strictly symptom-oriented behav-

Table 14. Acuteness of deviancy at close of therapy and follow-up

Frequency of behaviour	Therapy end (n=86)		Follow-up (n=51)	
	n	%	n	%
Highly acute	7	11	6	12
Frequently acute in crises	11	18	7	14
Seldom acute in crises	10	16	13	25
Only occasional phantasies	14	22	9	18
Not acute	21	33	16	31
Not assessable	23		0	
Total	86	100	51	100

Table 15. Changes in acuteness of deviancy at close of therapy and at follow-up relative to initial intensity

Assessment	Therapy end (n=86)		Follow-up (n=51)	
	n	%	n	%
Deteriorated	0	0	0	0
Unchanged	19	31	14	28
Slightly improved	8	13	7	14
Distinctly improved	14	22	13	25
Free of symptoms	21	33	16	31
Not assessable	24		1	
Total	86	99	51	98

iour therapy studies which report far better results: Maletzky (1980) reports on 155 exhibitionists who were treated with the indirectly aversive method of covert sensitization; 135 of the therapies were successful (almost 90%). Evans (1968, 1970) also reports higher success rates. We suspect that these higher success rates can be attributed to a different sample. For example: patients who cope ego-dystonically with their symptoms and have a pronounced need to punish themselves are certainly more willing to undergo aversive treatment. Accepting aversive methods of symptom control means, furthermore, submitting to the therapist to whom impulse control and superego functions are transferred, at least temporarily. The efficacy of aversive methods is linked extremely closely to the therapist's range of influence. In analogy to reports on therapy for alcoholism using aversive stimuli, we have the impression that aversively learnt impulse control tends to break down again in crises.

Our low therapy success rate is first of all a sign that our patients were far less carefully selected (see Sect. 2.1); furthermore, dropouts are included in our therapy sample for reasons we discussed in Sect. 2.1. Finally, the stability of our results at follow-up shows that our success rate is realistically assessed.

Changes in Social and Sexual Spheres

Table 16 illustrates social and occupational integration.

One third of the patients who had problems integrating socially, and a quarter who had employment difficulties at the start of therapy, had improved in this respect by the end of therapy - at follow-up the figure was even 50%-60%. This shows that the improvements could be maintained. Improvement in integration means, for instance, that patients had built up reliable social contacts and/or secured a steady job.

Table 17 shows the variable *sexual satisfaction* of the patients at the end of therapy and at follow-up.

Table 16. Social and occupational integration at close of therapy and at follow-up in comparison with start of therapy

Variable	Therapy end (n = 86)		Follow-up (n = 51)	
	n	%	n	%
Social integration				
Unremarkable before and after	14	19	6	13
Deteriorated	1	1	2	3
Still problematic	43	57	14	30
Slightly or distinctly improved	17	23	25	53
Not assessable	11		4	
Total	86	100	51	99
Occupational integration				
Unremarkable before and after	38	49	26	58
Deteriorated	1	1	1	2
Still problematic	29	38	7	16
Slightly or distinctly improved	9	12	11	24
Not assessable	9		6	
Total	86	100	51	100

Table 17. Sexual satisfaction at close of therapy and at follow-up in comparison with start of therapy

Sexual satisfaction	Therapy end (n = 86)		Follow-up (n = 51)	
	n	%	n	%
Unremarkable before and after	9	15	5	12
Deteriorated	–	–	–	–
Still problematic	30	48	18	44
Slightly or distinctly improved	23	37	18	44
Not assessable	24		10	
Total	86	100	51	100

The item sexual satisfaction combines various aspects. Sexual dissatisfaction can be the result of ungratified desire or a complete lack of erotic relationships, strong inhibitions, deep embarrassment and potency problems, or, on the other hand, the result of feeling that sexual impulses are compulsive and hard to keep under control. An increase in sexual satisfaction can therefore mean either that the patient's attitude to sexuality was less inhibited or embarrassed, that he had entered into a relationship or the quality of the relationship to his partner had improved, potency disorders had been surmounted or his sexuality was better integrated. The improvements here also stabilized in the period preceding follow-up.

The last aspect we should like to mention is our assessment of a *tendency towards depression*, the *alcohol problem* and *psychosomatic symptoms* (Table 18).

About half of the patients who had an alcohol problem were dry or had better control over alcohol consumption by the end of therapy. At follow-up this was true of three quarters of these patients. 60% of patients who had initially suffered from depressive symptoms had improved. This change was also stable at follow-up. However, little progress was made with psychosomatic symptoms.

We observed a symptom displacement in four patients. The following case is a striking example:

Case 3 (for previous history see p. 37)

Treatment of this patient lasted 2 years; his employer suggested therapy for his pedophile perversion which revealed sadistic and anal elements. In the first year weekly *individual behaviour therapy sessions* took place with a female therapist. He then joined *group therapy* for the second year.

In the first phase of therapy the therapist took on the role of a protective, understanding mother who amicably attended to the childlike, submissive patient. Owing to the pending trial and the symptoms he himself felt were a threat, the patient was under considerable pressure; consequently the therapist decided to start by concentrating on the symptom. She encouraged him when he carried out the self-control tasks and proudly reported on the outcome. In this affirmative mother-child arrangement the symptom became less acute and his self-confidence grew. Problems at work and with his parents could then be discussed. However, in this childishly dependent relationship with the maternal therapist, little progress was made on his interpersonal problems which arose from his inadequate grasp of reality, his poor ability to understand feelings and his paranoid coping. The therapy stagnated. For lack of any better idea, the therapist decided to take the patient into a group, in the hope that she could offer him a practice area, a protective space in which he could acquire new social competence. Being introduced to the group resulted in a reactivation of the patient's central trauma; he now had to share the "mother" with his siblings. He tried to cope with this situation by resorting to counterattack, dominating and attacking the group members, and so soon slipped back into the old outsider role. After a year of difficult therapeutic work, another problem arose: the therapist gave up work on the project as she was pregnant and handed over the group to another female therapist.

The patient's response to this double loss, initiated by the unwelcome siblings, was a *symptom displacement*. Although the perverse symptom faded into the background, a *colitis ulcerosa* developed which resulted in several stays in hospital. With this regressive somatization of the anal problem (autodestructive symptom formation), the aggressive and libidinous drives were redirected from phantasized and real objects onto his own body. As a kind of side effect, he now received the attention he yearned for on the anal level in the form of medical care (enemas, etc.).

Table 18. Alcohol problems, tendency towards depression and psychosomatic symptoms at the end of therapy and at follow-up in comparison with start of therapy

Variable	Therapy end (n=86)		Follow-up (n=51)	
	n	%	n	%
Alcohol problems				
Unremarkable before and after	47	60	30	67
Deteriorated	1	1	1	2
Still problematic	14	18	4	9
Slightly or distinctly improved	16	21	10	22
Not assessable	8		6	
Total	86	100	51	100
Tendency towards depression				
Unremarkable before and after	49	66	25	56
Deteriorated	–	–	–	–
Still problematic	9	12	9	20
Slightly or distinctly improved	16	22	11	24
Not assessable	12		6	
Total	86	100	51	100
Psychosomatic symptoms				
Unremarkable before and after	48	74	30	77
Deteriorated	2	3	2	5
Still problematic	12	18	6	15
Slightly or distinctly improved	3	5	1	3
Not assessable	21		12	
Total	86	100	51	100

During several phases of inpatient psychosomatic treatment the physical symptoms improved, but his perverse phantasies were reactivated several times. However, a perverse act has not occurred in the last 3 years. This is probably because the patient has turned to our department in times of crisis and "confessed" his phantasies, taking the pressure off himself. He turned down an offer of more regular sessions.

To summarize, in this case treatment did not do justice to the psychodynamics of the symptom. A reactivation of unsolved early loss experiences was probably responsible for the symptom displacement. However, the patient acquired a kind of first-aid kit during therapy: he is partly able to control the perverse symptom and uses the institute as his mainstay.

Once again, comparing these results with other studies is difficult because the criteria of success, if stated explicitly at all, vary greatly. Only Petri's (1980) investigation is at all comparable in terms of method. Petri arrived at a slightly more favourable evaluation of his patients' social and occupational situation and psychological stabilization. In Petri's investigation there was a tendency towards deterioration in the follow-ups which we did not observe. This effect may be due to the fact that Petri, as therapist, made the evaluations himself and perhaps tended towards a more favourable evaluation at the end of therapy. The differences are, however, only minor. Given the similarity, one can cautiously generalize that these results define the scope of what can presently be achieved with this kind of psychotherapeutic concept for sex offenders.

4.5.2.4 Overall Assessment of Therapy

A consensus was reached in the rater group by assessing each therapy on a six-point scale. This assessment is essentially intuitive and represents a consensus of subjective evaluations. In our discussions we did, however, use *guidelines* to help structure evaluations better. The following aspects served as guidelines:

- The quality and resilience of the therapist-patient relationship and changes in it during the therapeutic process.
- The choice of levels in the therapeutic approach (see Sect. 4.4.2) and their suitability to the patient's capabilities and limits. This is an assessment of how far a therapeutic gestalt developed and to what extent it coincided with the patient's problem. We also asked whether and to what extent the patient's central problem was recognized and actually dealt with in therapy.
- Changes in deviant symptoms; the focus was not only on whether and to what extent the symptoms had receded, but also on the patient's subjective feeling to what extent the impulses were under control and on changes in the patient's attitude towards them.
- Changes in the social sphere, covering assessment of the patient's ability to relate to others, his sex life and his social integration.
- Changes in neurotic symptom formation and his general state of mind.
- The stability of these changes until follow-up.

Altogether, it is important to emphasize that an overall assessment did not just include objective changes, but also covered the patient's subjective sense of wellbeing and satisfaction. As well as the degree of psychic health achieved in therapy, our assessment also included the limitations which the patient himself brings into the therapy (see the detailed discussion in the last section). This means we gauged what can be therapeutically achieved, given a specific starting-point.

The overall evaluation of therapies by the rater group using these criteria seems to us to be the most meaningful and valid statement on therapy outcome as it accounts for the patient's individual, overall problem and not merely separate and artificially isolated areas. The results of this assessment are shown in Table 19.

According to our assessment, one fifth of therapies were successful, two fifths were satisfactory and two fifths were inadequate. One should again remember that the relatively large number of unsuccessful therapies is due to the inclusion of therapy dropouts in the analysis (of 22 uncompleted therapies, 17 were rated inadequate). In Petri's investigation (1980), an overall evaluation of the therapies arrived at comparable results. Petri believes that a figure of 30% therapy success with "symptom removal and psychological and social restructuring" is realistic and probably reproducible. By combining his data for unsuccessful therapies and dropouts, one also arrives at a failure rate of about 40%.

The following is an example of a therapy assessed as successful (see also Case 10, p. 111; 14, p. 108).

Case 16 (see p. 70 for previous history)

After a 6-month prison sentence this patient was sent to us by court order for treatment as he had exposed himself to children. Treatment lasted 10 months with 25 sessions at weekly intervals.

The patient was distressed by deep self-contempt; he felt empty, lonely and resigned and tended more and more to take refuge in alcohol. During *conflict-oriented, client-centred therapy* a good working relationship developed and the patient increasingly opened up to the therapist, despite his initial resistance, fuelled by his recurring doubt whether he was really worth the effort. Therapy dealt mainly with his self-image as a failure and a "swine", his fear of being dependent and hemmed in combined with a tremendous, unadmitted longing for an intimate relationship. The patient became aware that his symptom's function was to help him escape from his tormenting loneliness and inner void. In the relationship to the therapist he felt respected and learnt to see himself in a more positive light; he understood that his symptom, which he had seen as expression of his depravity, was a call for help which the therapist had understood.

The patient expressed the wish to end therapy when he allowed himself a vacation for the first time. During the vacation he had several positive encounters and returned full of confidence. Although the therapist realized that the therapy had been terminated too soon, partly because of the patient's neurotic fear of dependency and intimacy, he respected his desire to retain his independence. Follow-up sessions showed that his self-confidence had stabilized in the course of 2½ years: he seldom drank alcohol, went on vacation regularly and was less morose at work. He had made friends with women, but had no steady relationship. Neither behaviour nor phantasies were deviant any longer.

To summarize, the patient's main experience in this relatively short therapy was that the therapist accepted him. This enabled him to demand less of himself and to accept himself

Table 19. Overall evaluation of therapies

Evaluation	n	%		
1. (Highly successful therapies)	2	2	17	59
2.	13	15		
3.	14	17	42	
4.	21	25		
5.	9	11	41	
6. (Failure)	24	30		
Not assessable	3			
Total	86	100		

more easily. This ego-supportive treatment, in which the patient also learnt to understand the function of his symptom, had apparently activated his constructive resources and reinforced his strengths. The therapeutic focus was well chosen, and the patient was healthy enough to place as much trust in the therapist as was needed for productive teamwork.

The following therapy was assessed as a failure because the patient's strategies of appeasement and problem minimization were not challenged and this prevented work on the real problem.

Case 18 (see p. 74 for previous history)

This patient had already undergone psychiatric examination several times; treatment took place during a 5-week stay in the University of Hamburg psychiatric clinic. The patient had been given "leave of absence" from a psychiatric state hospital in Southern Germany to which a court had committed him.

The hospital put us under considerable pressure to help him somehow therapeutically; as a result, we allowed ourselves to be persuaded to attempt a far too short-term therapy under unsatisfactory conditions. The patient had a severe structural disorder whose foremost problem was his almost complete lack of ability to control his destructive impulses and phantasies. As so often with patients showing symptoms of emotional neglect, he had acquired a certain skill in superficially adapting and functionalizing relationships. His fear of his destructive impulses was so strong that he resisted all attempts to discuss his offences. His desperate desire for love made him split off the "evil" aggressive side; consequently, he cooperated in exemplary fashion in behaviour therapy exercises which aimed at remedying his clumsiness in relating to others. His skill misled the therapist, who then overestimated the patient's ability to enter into relationships and unwittingly joined forces with him in denying the existence of his aggressive impulses. As a result, therapy failed. Only a few weeks after returning to the psychiatric state hospital a major relapse occurred.

We mentioned that overall assessment of therapy reflects not only objective improvements in the sense of psychic health, but also a patient's situation prior to therapy, his limitations and restricted ability to get involved in the therapeutic process. In other words, it is not only an assessment of what has been achieved, but also of what can be achieved. This in our view important aspect plays only a minor role in therapies which are clearly either successes or failures: therapies were only assessed as successful if deviant symptoms were no longer manifested or at least were no longer a danger. We considered therapy to have failed if no essential changes were seen in the symptoms and other problem areas. In therapies where there was partial success, however, this aspect is important. Among these patients we observed remarkable developments; therapy with severely disturbed patients helped them achieve an astonishing stability in everyday life in view of their pathology, even though one could not say they had been "cured" or their personality restructured. In this indeterminate area between success and failure, therapeutic work can be highly constructive. (see also Cases 4, p. 104; 12, p. 109). Here is an example:

Case 9 (see p. 50 for previous history)

This patient was admitted straight from prison to inpatient treatment, at first for 6 weeks, during which daily sessions took place with a female therapist. Outpatient treatment after this lasted 2 years with frequent sessions (2 to 3 per week), later with weekly sessions. In the first year the patient was given anti-androgen medication at his own request. The inpatient phase of treatment at first proved very difficult for the therapist as the patient was apprehensive, monosyllabic and unfriendly. He had no idea what the point of therapy was, but came to sessions regularly as he was afraid of being sent to a psychiatric institution. He only began to relax somewhat when the therapist organized *help in coping with his social circumstances* (work, money, apartment); this was the first time his everyday life gained some stability after many years of rootlessness and imprisonment.

Therapy was continued on an outpatient basis and with an additional male therapist. The latter's efforts to structure treatment and take a symptom-oriented approach were, however, permanently sabotaged by the patient. The therapist became an "evil persecutor" while the patient idealized the other therapist and allied himself closely with her. Motivated apparently by phantasies of rescuing the helpless and hopeless patient, she played the part of the yielding mother who successfully passed the patient's tolerance (love) tests. She also devoted time to him outside sessions, helped him plan his leisure time and make new contacts and encouraged him when he threatened to give up. Then with great difficulty he managed for the first time to talk about his sadistic phantasies; he was so shocked that he temporarily fell into a semistupor but was afterwards very relieved. In the course of therapy he began confiding his largely unrealistic plans to the therapist (for example, the plan to start a kindergarten or to learn Hebrew). They were carefully relativized and he made other plans which he was then partly able to put into practice. While the therapist was away on vacation a serious crisis and a relapse occurred; the patient fled in panic to Southern Germany where he wanted to commit suicide. The therapist persuaded him to return and join a self-help group where he met a woman with whom he had his first sexual contact without feeling he was a victim of his sadistic phantasies.

Since therapy began 8 years have passed. Apart from the one relapse, he has committed no further offence. The patient has a steady job, but lives in complete isolation, apart from occasional meetings with his therapist. In 1982 he asked to be hospitalized as he felt he was in danger of committing suicide; again, in a depressive crisis he turned to us. His sadistic phantasies continually recur, but they are no longer as compulsive.

To summarize, therapy was a highly complex "tight-rope walk". The patient's real problem was certainly not treated in therapy as he always resisted any such attempts. What helped him was a continuous relationship which gave him a minimum of security and a feeling for reality. The only chance for therapy was for the therapist not to give him up, but to help him survive.

4.5.2.5 Relapse Rate

Of the patients examined at follow-up 27% had again got into trouble with the law (charges brought and/or sentenced; Table 20). This corresponds to Petri's (1980) results (33% relapses). Other investigations quoted relapse rates below 20% (e.g. Conn 1949; Sachs 1965; Hacket 1971).

Table 20. Relapses at follow-up

	n	%
Yes	14	27
No	37	73
Total	51	100

4.5.2.6 Influence of Patient Variables on Therapy Results

We have correlated overall therapy evaluation, our most reliable criterion of success, with a number of variables.[7] We mention only the most important correlations.

Relationship Between Sexually Deviant Symptoms and Therapy Success

Table 21 shows the following tendency for the *acuteness of the deviancy*: the most favourable results were found in patients whose deviant desires only emerged in particular crises and where a sexual perversion was not a firmly established symptom. The relatively high percentage of unsuccessful therapies where the sexual deviancy was firmly established can be explained by the fact that a number of these patients (particularly some pedophiles) coped with and accepted the deviation ego-syntonically and tried to protect it from any therapeutic interference. This is also a sign that deviant orientation can be a deeply rooted conflict-solving pattern to which the patient can very quickly resort, making it extremely difficult to influence through therapy. The same point is illustrated by the fact that those patients whose therapy had an unsatisfactory outcome had significantly more often developed symptoms at an early stage in life – (late) puberty – compared with those patients where therapy outcome was good or medium ($p > 1\%$).

One important and, in theoretical terms, interesting result was that even patients whose symptoms became more severe in the sense of Giese's "sexual addiction" could be helped by psychotherapy without the assistance of anti-androgen medication. An increase in severity easily tempts one to imagine that a particularly vehement *vis naturalis* in the sense of powerful instinctual drives is at work here which, as it were, enforces its "own laws" (Rasch 1982) on the symptom both before and independently of any intrapsychic problem. The literature emphasizes that for these patients anti-androgens are indispensable as a prerequisite for therapy (Petri 1980). In successful therapies (cf. Case 10) it was impressive to see how the urgency and "untameability" of the perverse impulses vanished, often quite suddenly, as soon as the relationship with the therapist proved reliable and supportive.

There was no significant correlation between therapy outcome and the *type of sexual offence*.

Table 22 shows a possibly coincidental tendency: the outcome of therapy for indecent exposure to adult women was frequently assessed more positively than pedophile offences and rape. However, we should like to stress that psychotherapy can be indicated and even successful with sex offenders in general,

---

[7] Correlations were calculated for a maximum of 62 of the 86 patients; we excluded 24 patients whose previous history and therapy record were insufficiently documented to avoid blurring correlations. In view of the small sample numbers in each field we dispensed with percent figures. Significance calculated using the chi-square test is slightly uncertain in view of the small cell frequency.

Table 21. Therapy evaluation (contingency coefficient C = 0.34, significance p = 10.1%)

Intensity of sexual deviancy	Good	Medium	Poor	Total
Deviancy not firmly established	6	4	2	12
Firmly established, no increase in severity	4	16	14	34
Increase in severity	4	6	5	15
Total	14	26	21	61

Table 22. Relationship between therapy evaluation and type of sex offence (contingency coefficient C = 0.24, significance p = 73.7%)

Type of sex offence	Therapy evaluation			
	Good	Medium	Poor	Total
Indecent exposure to children	2	8	6	16
Indecent exposure to women	5	6	3	14
Sexual acts with children	4	7	8	19
Rape/sexual molestation	2	3	4	9
Total	13	24	21	58

irrespective of the kind of offence. The forensic definition of an illness usually also implies a criminalistic judgement, in that therapy is more likely to be considered for socially less harmful acts than for violent offences which are dealt with more as a matter for prosecution and public safety (see, for example, Horn, 1971). It is therefore no coincidence that the law is interpreted in such a way that psychotherapeutic treatment is only considered as an alternative when the offence is indecent exposure to women, but not for indecent exposure to children, which is assessed differently legally although the underlying problems are similar. This kind of distinction does not fit in with therapeutic thinking and practice which show that, on the contrary, particularly aggressive impulses can be a sign of decompensation in a crisis (see Case 5, p. 90).

A similar, but not significant tendency emerges if one disregards the legal definition of a crime and instead distinguishes between violent and nonviolent acts (Table 23).

It is commonly believed that psychotherapy is only possible if it is strictly voluntary. Many patients ordered by a court to seek therapy are rejected for this reason. This basic assumption stems from experience with the traditional psychotherapeutic clientele. When projected onto groups of social outsiders, such as delinquents, it ignores their actual circumstances. In our study a comparison between patients sent by *court order* and those who were not revealed no difference. A court order is by no means an argument against therapy (Table 24). We refer the reader to Sect. 4.2 in which we demonstrated how important it is to take account of pretherapy circumstances and the often real objective difficulties affecting motivation for therapy.

Table 23. Relationship between therapy evaluation and use of violence by offenders (contingency coefficient C = 0.25, significance p = 12.7%)

Violence	Therapy evaluation			
	Good	Medium	Poor	Total
Yes	6	5	9	20
No	8	21	11	40
Total	14	26	20	60

Table 24. Relationship between therapy evaluation and court order/pending trial (contingency coefficient C = 0.15, significance p = 51.9%)

Court order/pending trial	Therapy evaluation			
	Good	Medium	Poor	Total
Yes	5	16	11	32
No	7	10	9	26
Total	12	26	20	58

Relationship Between Social Status and Therapy Outcome

Attempts were made in the early days of psychotherapy to avoid focussing exclusively on the middle and upper classes and make it available to minority groups (for example, Aichhorn 1935; see alse the survey in Böllinger 1979). Extending the horizon forces one to modify the prerequisites associated with the middle classes such as intelligence, introspective ability, distress and motivation for therapy. This is discussed in Sect. 4.2. When evaluating the therapies no significant differences were found relating to social class. Although there is a tendency for therapy with lower-class patients to be less successful, this is probably due to other factors such as social instability and severe personality disorders, which were more frequent in the lower-class patients in our sample (Table 25).

Relationship Between Personality Structure and Therapy Outcome

We restrict ourselves here mainly to the correlations between therapy evaluation and the groups formed by cluster analysis (see Sect. 3.6; Table 26).

The distribution shows an important, though nonsignificant tendency. The correlations were as follows: the best therapy results were not found, as might be expected, in cluster 1 (psychically stable, apparently healthiest and socially well-integrated patients), but in cluster 2 - depressive patients who, unlike those in clusters 1 and 3, feel they need and are dependent on help and are therefore more open to a therapeutic relationship. The most difficult group is cluster 5 (severely disturbed patients without social ties). The difficulties here

Table 25. Relationship between therapy evaluation and social class (contingency coefficient C = 0.25, significance p = 16.2%)

Social class	Therapy evaluation			
	Good	Medium	Poor	Total
Middle class	6	16	4	26
Lower class	6	13	14	33
Total	12	29	18	59

Table 26. Relationship between therapy evaluation and cluster analysis groups (contingency coefficient C = 0.45, significance p = 6.5%)

Patient group	Therapy evaluation			
	Good	Medium	Poor	Total
Cluster 1: psychically more stable socially integrated	3	8	2	13
Cluster 2: depressive tendencies	6	5	2	13
Cluster 3: patients with marked defences against depression	1	4	2	7
Cluster 4: (not interpretable)	1	6	5	12
Cluster 5: severely disturbed, social outsiders	2	3	9	14
Total	13	26	20	59

are even clearer if one looks at individual correlations: the significant correlation between therapy outcome and lack of social integration ($p < 1\%$; $C = 0.43$) or severe personality pathology ($p < 1\%$; $C = 0.42$). These correlations are not surprising. They are frequently found in psychotherapy and were also observed in the survey by Luborsky et al. (1971) who analysed which factors influenced therapy outcome in 166 psychotherapeutic studies made between 1946 and 1969. Here, too, we should like to emphasize that there is no justification for the prejudices that arise out of such correlations; almost one third of the patients in cluster 5 had some kind of success in therapy and in 2 of the 14 cases therapy was rated a success.

Relationship Between Special Aspects of Therapy and Therapy Outcome

The highly significant correlation between the quality of the patient-therapist relationship and therapy outcome is an important, though hardly surprising result ($C = 0.69$). We were particularly struck by another result. In Sect. 4.4.2 we distinguished between four levels of therapeutic approach: practical everyday help, crisis intervention (these two are combined in Table 27), current behaviour and feelings and interpretation of emotional contexts. We explained that there is no difference in importance between the four levels and that, in fact, they should be seen as equal since the choice of level depends less on the therapist's training than on the given abilities and limitations of the patient. Table 27 shows that there are no significant differences in therapy outcome here. The tendency towards a poorer result with everyday help and crisis intervention can be attributed to the fact that levels one and two were combined owing to low cell frequency and that therapies which were essentially restricted to help with everyday life were assessed as inadequate.

Table 27. Relationship between therapy evaluation and level of therapy approach (contingency coefficient $C = 0.29$, significance $p = 31.5\%$)

Level of approach	Therapy evaluation			
	Good	Medium	Poor	Total
Help in coping with everyday life and current crisis	2	4	5	11
Level of actual behaviour and feelings	7	12	10	29
Interpretation of emotional contexts	5	7	1	13
Total	14	23	16	53

5 Conclusions and Perspectives for Patient Welfare

Even when examined critically, our results allow us to conclude that outpatient psychotherapy can be successfully conducted with over 50% of sex offenders. This is encouraging considering the marked scepticism towards psychotherapy shown not only by the legal authorities, but also by psychotherapists who doubt whether psychotherapy can be effective in criminal delinquents, especially if they have perverse symptoms. The success rate would increase considerably if one used narrower selection criteria than ours. This was not our intention; we wanted to include a broad spectrum and to evaluate to what extent psychotherapy is suitable for these patients. In retrospect we are glad we did not restrict ourselves by using standard selection criteria as with our therapy approach we succeeded in working with patients who are otherwise considered virtually beyond the reach of therapy. Another important outcome of our study is that it provides criteria for a differentiated indication within a flexible therapeutic procedure.

Our work also showed that psychotherapy for sexual delinquents is not essentially a problem for specialists. Although we do not mean to overlook and in fact have always stressed the uniqueness of the situation - perverse symptoms, on the one hand, and the conflict with the law and its enforcement, on the other - this kind of therapy forms a part of psychotherapy's overall responsibility. In view of the growing tendency amongst therapists to propagate more and more "special therapies" for more and more "special disorders" (especially in so-called sex therapy), it is always worth emphasizing the obvious fact that there is, and can be, no "special programme" for sexual delinquents. The call for a specialist in this field is always a sign of fear of getting involved with these patients - a fear which our project among other things aimed at reducing.

Our rather eclectic therapeutic approach seems to have stood up to the test. Our results show that very different therapeutic methods can be successfully implemented, provided the therapist understands the psychodynamics and always takes into account the function and significance of the perverse symptoms. We hope our book will inspire and encourage therapists from various schools of thought to devote attention to this problem group.

Financing therapy research is often linked to absurdities in the health care situation with which we too had to contend: at the beginning of the project we publicized the fact that therapy was now available for these patients. Over the years it became common practice for the courts, lawyers and probation officers to send us patients who we included in the therapy project. When our financial resources dried up this constructive cooperation collapsed for lack of therapy places and we were left with guilty consciences for no longer being able to take over the responsiblity we had once offered. This was a dilemma - the result of the division between research and health care - we were not prepared to tolerate. Consequently, we continued to seek ways of putting our research results into practice in health care.

The lack of funds had one positive side effect; there was no longer an institution available specialized in the treatment of sexual delinquents. The advantage was a psychological one, since a central institution encourages an uncritical belief in specialists. In our opinion, *decentralized care* for these patients would make much more sense; regional therapists and therapeutic institutions should feel responsible and offer treatment. This model has other advantages over a specialized institution: a "centre for the treatment of sexual delinquents" would involve a greater risk of stigmatizing patients and increasing their fear of getting in touch. Moreover, the necessarily close cooperation between the judiciary, prison authorities and an institution of this kind could give a patient the impression that the institutions are too closely interwoven and so handicap psychotherapy. Finally, our experience in the project has taught us that it is inadvisable to restrict therapists to treating sexual delinquents only as this can be overdemanding and restrict perspectives.

Consequently, the therapists still available after completing the project only provide psychotherapy for individuals on a limited scale; we invest most of our energy in encouraging existing psychotherapeutic institutes to offer therapy. We have written to psychotherapists, organized training seminars and offer continuous supervision, individually and in groups, for therapists treating these patients. We have been at least modestly successful in interesting more therapists.

We are aware that our experience with outpatient therapy can do little to solve the therapeutic dilemma of these patients in prisons, psychiatric clinics and homes. Each institution has its own individual structures which create specific therapeutic problems. However, during group supervision for the staff from these institutions we found that our diagnostic and therapeutic concept has helped them, even though the therapeutic procedure cannot be applied identically. We believe our project has succeeded in contributing to the groundwork needed for making psychotherapy available to patients in other institutions.

References

Abel GG, Leavis DJ, Clancy J (1970) Aversion therapy applied to taped sequences of deviant behaviour in exhibitionism and other sexual deviations. J Behav Ther Exp Psychiatry 1: 59

Abel GG, Blanchard EB, Jackson M (1974) The role of fantasy in the treatment of sexual deviation. Arch Gen Psychiatry 30: 467

Abel GG, Blanchard EB, Becker JV (1978) An integrated treatment program for rapists. In: Rada ED (ed) Clinical aspects of the rapist. Grune & Stratton, New York, p 161

Aichhorn A (1935) Wayward youth. Viking, New York

Alford GS, Webster JS, Sanders SH (1980) Covert aversion of two interrelated deviant sexual practices: Obscene phonecalling and exhibitionism. A single case analysis. Behav Res Ther 11: 15

Appel JB (1964) Analysis of aversively motivated behavior. Arch Gen Psychiatry 10: 71

Appelbaum A (1972) A critical re-examination of the concept "motivation for change" in psychoanalytic treatment. Int J Psychoanal 53: 51

Arentewicz G, Schmidt G (eds) (1983) The treatment of sexual disorders - concept and techniques of couple therapy. Basic Books, New York

Baekeland F, Lundwall L (1975) Dropping out of treatment: A critical review. Psychol Bull 82: 738

Bak RC (1953) Fetishism. J Am Psychoanal Assoc 1: 285

Bak RC (1971) Object-relationship in schizophrenia and perversion. Int J Psychoanal 52: 235

Balint M (1952a) On love and hate. Int J Psychoanal 33: 355-362

Balint M (1952b) Primary love and psychoanalytic treatment. Tavistock, London

Bancroft J (1974) Deviant sexual behavior modification and assessment. Clarendon, Oxford

Bancroft J (1979) The nature of the patient-therapist relationship. Br J Criminol 19: 416

Bancroft J (1983) Human sexuality and its problems. Livingstone, London

Bandura A (1962) Punishment revisted. J Consult Psychol 26: 298

Bandura A (1969) Principles of behavior modification. Holt, Rinehart & Winston, New York

Bandura A, Walters RH (1963) Social learning and personality development. Holt, Rinehart & Winston, New York

Barlow DH (1973) Increasing heterosexual responsiveness in the treatment of sexual deviation: A review of the clinical and experimental literature. Behav Res Ther 4: 655

Barlow DH (1974) The treatment of sexual deviation: Toward a comprehensive behavioral approach. In: Calhoun KS, Adams HE, Mitchell KM (eds) Innovative treatment methods in psycho-pathology. Wiley, New York

Barlow DH, Abel GG (1976) Sexual deviation. In: Craighead WE, Kazdin AE, Mahoney MG (eds) Behavior modification: Principles, issues and applications. Houghton Mifflin, Boston

Barlow DH, Leitenberg H, Agras WS (1969) Experimental control of sexual deviation through manipulation of the noxious scene in covert sensitization. J Abnorm Psychol 74: 597

Becker JV, Abel GG, Blanchard EB, Murphy WD, Coleman E (1978) Evaluating social skills of sexual aggressives. Criminal Justice Behav 5: 357

Becker N, Schorsch E (1980) Die psychoanalytische Theorie sexueller Perversionen. In: Sigusch V (Hrsg) Therapie sexueller Störungen, 2. Aufl. Thieme, Stuttgart, S 159

Beech HR, Watts F, Poole AD (1971) Classical conditioning of sexual deviation - preliminary note. Behav Ther 2: 213-216

Bergmann MS (1971) Psychoanalytic observations on the capacity to love. In: McDevitt IB, Settlage CF (eds) Separation - Individuation. Int Univ Press, New York
Blair DC, Lanyon RI (1981) Exhibitionism: Etiology and treatment. Psychol Bull 89: 439
Blakemore CB et al. (1963) The application of faradic aversion conditioning in a case of transvestitism. Behav Res Ther 1: 29
Blanck G, Blanck R (1974) Ego psychology: theory and practice. Columbia University Press, New York
Böllinger L (1979) Psychoanalyse und die Behandlung von Delinquenten. Müller, Heidelberg Karlsruhe
Bond IK, Evans DR (1967) Avoidance therapy: Its use in two cases of underwear fetishism. Can Med Assoc J 96: 1160
Bond IK, Hutchinson HC (1964) Application of reciprocal inhibition therapy to exhibitionism. In: Eysenck HJ (ed) Experiments in behaviour therapy. Pergamon, Oxford
Boudreau L et al. (1978) Multiple behaviour therapy techniques applied to a case of forcible sexual assault. J Behav Ther Exp Psychiatry 9: 335
Boudwyns PA, Tanna VL, Fleischmann DJ (1975) A modified shame aversion therapy for compulsive obscene telephone calling. Behav Res Ther 6: 704
Bräutigam W (1966) Indikation und Prognose bei analytisch nicht behandelbaren Krankheitsbildern. Z Psychother Med Psychol 16: 105
Brecher EM (1978) Treatment programs for sex offenders. National institute of law enforcement and criminal justice. Law enforcement assistance administration. US Department of Justice, Washington
Brodsky SL, West DJ (1981) Life-skills treatment of sex offenders. Law Psychol Rev 6: 97
Bronisch T (1983) Auswirkungen neuerer psychoanalytischer Theorien und Therapiekonzepte auf die Behandlungstechnik von Sexualdelinquenten. Psychiatr Prax 10: 75
Bronisch T, Berger M, Kockott G (1983) Integratives Therapiekonzept bei stationärer Behandlung von Sexualdelinquenten. Psychiatr Prax 10: 83
Brownell KD, Barlow DH (1976) Measurement and treatment of two sexual deviations in one person. J Behav Exp Psychiatry 7: 349
Brownell KD, Barlow DH (1977) Pattern of appropriate and deviant sexual arousal: The behavioural treatment of multiple sexual deviations. J Consult Clin Psychol 45: 1144
Burdick MR (1972) An exploration of the aversion therapie technique of covert sensitization with selected cases of exhibitionism. Diss Abs Intern 33: 2805
Callahan EJ, Leitenberg H (1973) Aversion therapy for sexual deviation. Contingent shock and covert sensitization. J Abnorm Psychol 81: 60
Cartwright D, Roth I (1957) Success and satisfaction in psychotherapy. J Clin Psychol 13: 20
Cautela JR, Wisocki PA (1971) Covert sensitization for the treatment of sexual deviations. Psychol Res 21: 37
Clark DF (1965) A note on avoidance conditioning techniques in sexual disorders. Behav Res Ther 3: 203
Conn H (1949) Brief psychotherapy of the sex offenders. J Clin Psychopathol 10: 347
Conrad SR, Wince JP (1976) Orgasmic reconditioning: A controlled study of its effects upon the sexual arousal and behavior of adult male homosexuals. Behav Res Ther 7: 155
Cooper AJ (1963) A case of fetishism and impotence treated by behavior modification. Br J Psychiatry 109: 649
Crawford DA (1979) Modification of deviant sexual behaviour: The need for a comprehensive approach. Br J Med Psychol 52: 151
Crawford DA, Allen JV (1979) A social skills training program with sex offenders. In: Cook M, Wilson G (eds) Love and attraction. Pergamon, Oxford, p 503
Dahl H (1972) A quantitative study of psychoanalysis. In: Holt RR, Peterfreund E (eds) Psychoanalysis and contemporary science. McMillan, New York
Das Argument 60 (1970) Kritik der bürgerlichen Medizin. Argument, Berlin
Das Argument 71 (1972) Argument für eine soziale Medizin (III). Argument, Berlin
Das Argument 78 (1973) Argumente für eine soziale Medizin (IV). Argument, Berlin
Das Argument 89 (1975) Argumente für eine soziale Medizin (VI). Argument, Berlin

Davis BF, Morgenstern A (1960) A case of cysticercosis, temporal lobe epilepsy, and transvestitism. J Neurol Neurosurg Psychiatry 23: 247
Davison GC (1968) Elimination of sadistic fantasy by a client-controlled counterconditioning technique: A case study. J Abnorm Psychol 73: 84
Dengrove E (1967) Behavior therapy of the sexual disorders. J Sex Res 3: 49
Dummer W, Burian DR (1978) Ein Behandlungskonzept für sexuelle Deviationen (Methodik und bisherige Ergebnisse). Psychiatr Neurol Med Psychol (Leipz) 30: 599
Edwards NB (1972) Case conference. Assertive training in a case of homosexual pedophilia. J Behav Ther Exp Psychiatry 3: 55
Eidelberg L (1958) Über die innere und äußere narzißtische Kränkung. Psyche (Stuttg) 11: 672
Eissler KR (1958) Notes on problems of technique in the psychoanalytic treatment of adolescents. With some remarks on perversions. Psychoanal Study Child 13: 223-254
Evans DR (1967) An exploratory study into the treatment of exhibitionism by means of emotive imagery and aversive conditioning. Can J Psychol 8: 162
Evans DR (1968) Masturbatory fantasy and sexual deviation. Behav Res Ther 6: 17
Evans DR (1970) Subjective variables and treatment effects in aversion therapy. Behav Res Ther 8: 147
Feldmann MP, McCulloch MJ, McCulloch ML (1968) The aversion therapy treatment of a heterogenous group of five cases of sexual deviation. Acta Psychiatr Scand 44: 113
Fenichel O (1932) Spezielle psychoanalytische Neurosenlehre. Internationaler Psychoanalytischer Verlag, Wien
Fensterheim H (1974) Behaviour therapy of sexual variations. J Sex Marital Ther 1: 16
Fookes BH (1969) Some experiences in the use of aversion therapy in male homosexuality, exhibitionism and fetishism-transvestitism. Br J Psychiatry 115: 339
Foot WE, Laws DR (1981) A daily alternation procedure for orgasmic reconditioning with a pedophile. J Behav Ther Exp Psychiatry 12: 267
Freud A (1937) The ego and the mechanisms of defence. Hogarth, London
Freud S (1905) Three essays on the theory of sexuality. SE vol VII
Freud S (1919) 'A child is being beaten'. SE vol XVII
Freud S (1927) Fetishism. SE vol XXI
Freud S (1938) Splitting of the ego in process of defence. SE vol XXIII
Fülgraff G, Barbey I (1978) Stereotaktische Hirnoperationen bei abweichendem Sexualverhalten. Abschlußbericht der Kommission beim Bundesgesundheitsamt. (bga-Berichte 3/1978), Reimer, Berlin
Fürstenau P (1977) Die beiden Dimensionen des psychoanalytischen Umgangs mit strukturell ich-gestörten Patienten. Psyche (Stuttg) 3: 197
Gaupp LA et al. (1971) The use of aversion relief procedures in the treatment of a case of voyeurism. Behav Res Ther 2: 585
Gershman L (1970) Case Conference: A transvestite fantasy treated by thoughtstopping, covert sensitization and aversive shock. J Behav Ther Exp Psychiatry 1: 153
Giese H (1962) Psychopathologie der Sexualität. Enke, Stuttgart
Giese U, Kober EM (1983) Ambulante Gruppentherapie mit Sexualdelinquenten. Psychiatr Prax 10: 88
Glick BS (1972) Aversive imagery therapy using hypnosis. Am J Psychother 26: 432
Glover E (1956) The relation of perversion-formation to the development of reality-sense. In: Glover E (ed) On the early development of the mind. International Universities Press, New York
Goldberg A (1975) A fresh look at perverse behavior. Int J Psychoanal 56: 335
Goudsmit W, Reicher JW (1980) Sozialtherapie schwerstgestörter Delinquenten auf psychoanalytischer Grundlage. In: Sigusch V (Hrsg) Therapie sexueller Störungen. Thieme, Stuttgart
Grawe K, Dziewas H (1977) Interaktionelle Verhaltenstherapie. Partnerberatung 14: 188
Greenacre P (1952) Trauma, growth and personality. Int Univ Press, New York
Greenacre P (1953) Certain relationships between fetishism and the faulty development of the body image: Psychoanal Study Child 8: 79
Greenacre P (1955) Further considerations regarding fetishism. Psychoanal Study Child 10: 187

Greenacre P (1960) Further notes on fetishism. Psychoanal Study Child 15: 187
Greenacre P (1968) Perversions: General considerations regarding their genetic and dynamic background. Psychoanal Study Child 23: 47
Greenson RR (1961/62) Zum Problem der Empathie. Psyche (Stuttg) 15: 142
Gretenkord L (1981) Mehrdimensionale Therapie eines Sexualdelinquenten in einer forensischen Klinik. Monatsschr Kriminol 64: 353
Groth AN (1979) Men who rape. The psychology of the offender. Plenum, New York London
Guilford JP (1954) Psychometric methods, 2nd edn. McGraw-Hill, New York
Haag A (1980) Zur Problematik der psychoanalytischen Behandlung sexueller Deviationen mit besonderer Berücksichtigung sexueller Straftäter. Materialien zur Psychoanalyse und analytisch orientierten Psychotherapie 4: 243
Hackett T (1971) The psychotherapy of exhibitionists in a court clinic setting. Semin Psychiatry 3: 297
Harbert TL et al. (1974) Measurement and modification of incestous behaviour: A case study. Psychol Rep 34: 79
Hayes SC, Brownell KD, Barlow DH (1978) The use of self-administrated covert sensitization in a case of multiple sexual deviation. Behav Res Ther 9: 283
Heim N (1977) Kastration bei Sexualstraftätern - eine kritische Betrachtung. In: Nass G (Hrsg) Kriminalätiologie und Prophylaxe. Abhandlungen der Akademie für kriminologische Grundlagenforschung (5. Folge). Verlag Gesellschaft für vorbeugende Verbrechensbekämpfung, Kassel
Herman SH et al. (1974) An experimental analysis of exposure to explicit heterosexual stimuli as an effective variable in changing arousal patterns of homosexuals. Behav Res Ther 12: 335
Horn HF (1971) Der Leidensdruck als Indikationskriterium. Bemerkungen zur "medikamentösen Kastration". Nervenarzt 42: 312
Horn HJ (1974) Administration of antiandrogens in hypersexuality and sexual deviations. In: Eichler O, Farah A, Herken H, Welch AD (eds) Androgens II and antiandrogens. Springer, Berlin Heidelberg New York (Handbook of experimental pharmacology, vol 35/2)
Hughes RC (1977) Covert sensitization treatment of exhibitionism. J Behav Ther Exp Psychiatry 8: 177
Jacobson E (1973) The self and the object world. Int Univ Press, New York
Jessen JL (1969) Behandlungsresultate in der Van der Hoeven Klinik. Ned Tijdschr Criminol 11: 173
Jones IH, Frei D (1977) Provoked anxiety as a treatment of exhibitionism. Br J Psychiatry 131: 295
Josiassen RC, Fantuzzo J, Rosen AC (1980) Treatment of pedophilia using multistage aversion therapy and social skills training. J Behav Ther Exp Psychiatry 11: 55
Kächele H, Schors R (1981) Ansätze und Ergebnisse psychoanalytischer Therapieforschung. In: Baumann U, Berbalk H, Seidenstücker G (Hrsg) Klinische Psychologie, Trends in Forschung und Praxis. Huber, Bern
Kanfer FH (1977) Selbstmanagement-Methoden. In: Kanfer FH, Goldstein AP (Hrsg) Möglichkeiten der Verhaltensänderung. Urban & Schwarzenberg, München
Keltner A, Scharf N, Schell R (1978) The assessment and training of assertive skills with sexuell offenders. Correct Soc Psychiatry Behav Technol Ther 24: 88
Kernberg OF (1975) Borderline conditions and pathological narcissism. Aronson, New York
Kernberg OF (1976) Object relations theory and clinical psychoanalysis. Aronson, New York
Khan MMR (1979) Alienation in perversions. Hogarth and The Institute of Psychoanalysis, London
Klein M (1932) Psychoanalysis of children. Hogarth, London
Kockott G (Hrsg) (1977) Sexuelle Störungen. Urban & Schwarzenberg, München
Kockott G (1983) Verhaltenstherapie bei sexuellen Deviationen - ein orientierender Überblick. Psychiatr Prax 10: 78
Kohlenberg RJ (1974) Treatment of a homosexual pedophiliac using in vivo desensitization: A case study. J Abnorm Soc Psychol 83: 192

Kohut H (1973a) Überlegungen zum Narzißmus und zur narzißtischen Wut. Psyche (Stuttg) 6: 513
Kohut H (1973b) The analysis of the self. A systematic approach to the psychoanalytic treatment of narcisstic personality disorders. Int Univ Press, New York
Kolvin L (1967) "Aversive imagery" treatment in adolescents. Behav Res Ther 5: 245
Kremsdorf RB et al. (1980) Orgasmic reconditioning without deviant imagery: A case report with a pedophile. Behav Res Ther 18: 203
Kurlychek RT (1978) Cognitive perspective therapy in the treatment of sexual offenders. Correct Soc Psychiatr J Behav Technol Methods Ther 26: 29
Kursbuch 28 (1972a) Das Elend mit der Psychiatrie I. Psychiatrie. Kursbuch-Verlag, Berlin
Kursbuch 29 (1972b) Das Elend mit der Psychiatrie II. Psychoanalyse. Kursbuch-Verlag, Berlin
Lande SD (1980) A combination of orgasmic reconditioning and covert sensitization in the treatment of a fire fetish. Behav Ther Exp Psychiatry 11: 291
Langelüddeke A (1963) Die Entmannung von Sittlichkeitsverbrechern. deGruyter, Berlin
Langevin R, Paitich D, Hucker S et al. (1979) The effect of assertiveness training, provera and sex of therapist in the treatment of genital exhibitionism. Behav Ther Exp Psychiatry 10: 275
Laws DR (1980) Treatment of bisexual pedophilia by a biofeedback-assisted selfcontrol procedure. Behav Res Ther 18: 207
Lazarus AA (1967) In support of technical electicism. Psychol Rep 21: 415
Lazarus AA (1976) Multimodal behavior therapy. Springer, Berlin Heidelberg New York
Levin SM, Barry SM, Gambaro S, Wolfinsohn L, Smith A (1977) Variations of covert sensitization in the treatment of pedophilic behaviour: A case study. J Consult Clin Psychol 45: 896
Lichtenstein H (1961) Identity and sexuality. J Am Psychoanal Assoc 9: 179
Lichtenstein H (1970) Changing implications of the concept of psychosexual development. J Am Psychoanal Assoc 18: 300
Luborsky L (1962) The patient's personality and psychotherapeutic change. In: Strupp H, Luborsky H (eds) Research in psychotherapy, vol 2. American Psychological Association, Washington
Luborsky L, Spence DP (1978) Quantitative research on psychoanalytic therapy. In: Garfield S, Bargin AE (eds) Handbook of psychotherapy and behavior change. Wiley, New York
Luborsky L, Chandler M, Auerbach AH, Cohen J (1971) Factors influencing the outcome of psychotherapy: A review of quantitative research. Psychol Bull 75: 145
Mahler MS (1975) The psychological birth of the human infant. Basic Books, New York
Maletzky BM (1974) Assisted covert sensitization in the treatment of exhibitionism. J Consult Clin Psychol 42: 34
Maletzky BM (1977) Booster sessions in aversion therapy: The permancy of treatment. Behav Res Ther 8: 460
Maletzky BM (1980) Assisted covert sensitization. In: Cox OJ, Daitzman RJ (eds) Exhibitionism: Description, assessment and treatment. Garland, New York
Marks IM, Gelder M (1967) Transvestism and fetishism. Clinical and psychological changes during faradic aversion. Br J Psychiatry 113: 711
Marks IM, Rachman S, Gelder MG (1965) Methods for assessment of aversion treatment in fetishism with masochism. Behav Res Ther 3: 253
Marquis JN (1970) Orgasmic reconditioning: Changing sexual object choice through controlling the masturbation fantasies. J Behav Ther Exp Psychiatry 1: 263
Marshall WL (1971) A combined treatment method for certain sexual deviations. Behav Res Ther 9: 293
Marshall WL (1973) The modification of sexual fantasies: A combined treatment approach to the reduction of deviant behavior. Behav Res Ther 11: 557
Marshall WL (1974) A combined treatment approach to the reduction of multiple fetish-related behaviors. J Consult Clin Psychol 42: 613
Marshall WL (1979) Satiation therapy: A procedure for reducing deviant sexual arousal. J Appl Behav Anal 12: 377

Marshall WL, Barbarec HE (1978) The reduction of deviant arousal satiation treatment for sexual aggressors. Criminal Justice Behav 5: 294
Marshall WL, Lippens K (1977) The clinical value of boredom. J Nerv Ment Dis 165: 283
Marshall WL, McKnight RD (1975) An integrated treatment program for sexual offenders. Can Psychiatry Assoc J 20: 133
Masters W, Johnson V (1970) Human sexual inadequacy. Little Brown, Boston
Mathis HJ (1975) Instating sexual adequacy in a disabled exhibitionist. Psychother Theory Res Pract 12: 97
Mathis JL, Collins M (1970) Progressive phases in the group therapy of exhibitionists. Int J Group Psychother 20: 163
McCulloch MJ, Williams C, Birtles CJ (1971) The successful application of aversion therapy to an adolescent exhibitionist. J Behav Ther Exp Psychiatry 2: 61
McGark BJ, Newell TC (1981) Social skills training with a sex offender. Psychol Record 31: 277
McGuire RJ, Carlisle JM, Young BG (1977) Sexual deviations as conditional behaviour: A hypothesis. Behav Res Ther 2: 185-190
McKay D (1976) Modification of sexual behavior. In: Crown G (ed) Psychosexual problems: Psychotherapy, counselling and behavior modification. Academic Press, London
Mentzos S (1982) Neurotische Konfliktverarbeitung. Kindler, München
Metzner R (1963) Some experimental analogous of obsession. Behav Res Ther 1: 231
Meyer AE (1981) The Hamburg short psychotherapy comparison experiment. In: Meyer AE (ed) Psychotherapy and psychosomatics. Karger, Basel München Paris London New York Sidney
Miller HL, Haney JR (1976) Behavior and traditional therapy applied to pedophiliac exhibitionism: A case study. Psychol Rep 39: 1119
Mintz J (1972) What is "success" in psychotherapy? J Abnorm Psychol 80: 11
Mohr JW (1971) Evaluation of treatment. Int Psychol Clin 4: 227
Morgenthaler F (1974) Die Stellung der Perversionen in Metapsychologie und Technik. Psyche (Stuttg) 28: 1077
Morgenthaler F (1984) Sexualität und Psychoanalyse. Beitr Sexualforsch 59: 20
Moser T (1972) Jugendkriminalität und Gesellschaftsstruktur. Fischer, Frankfurt
Neumann FH, Steinbeck H (1974) Antiandrogens. In: Eichler O, Farah A, Herken H, Welch AD (eds) Androgens II and antiandrogens. Springer, Berlin Heidelberg New York (Handbook of experimental pharmacology, vol 35/2)
Nolan JD, Sandman C (1978) "Biosyntonic" therapy: Modification of an operant conditioning approach to pedophilia. J Consult Clin Psychol 46: 1133
Petri H (1980) Analytische Kurztherapie bei sexuellen Perversionen. In: Sigusch V (Hrsg) Therapie sexueller Störungen, 2. Aufl. Thieme, Stuttgart, S 187
Pinard G, Lamontagne Y (1976) Electrical aversion relief and sexual retraining in the treatment of fetishism with masochism. J Behav Ther Exp Psychiatry 7: 71
Ploog D, Bronisch T, Berger U, Kockott G (1982) Stationäre Psychotherapie von Sexualdelinquenten unter Einbeziehung verhaltenstherapeutischer Verfahren. Partnerberatung 19: 12
Pohlen M, Wittmann L (1983) Die Modernisierung der Verhaltenstherapie. Psyche (Stuttg) 37: 961
Powell J, Azrin N (1968) The effects of shock as a punisher for cigarette smoking. J Appl Behav Anal 1: 63
Quinsey VL, Chaplin TC, Carrigan WF (1980) Biofeedback and signaled punishment in the modification of inappropriate sexual age preverences. Behav Res Ther 11: 567
Rachman S (1966) Sexual fetishism: An experimental analogue. Psychol Rec 16: 293-296
Rachman S, Hodgson RJ (1969) Experimentally induced sexual fetishism, replication and development. Psychol Rec 18: 25-27
Rachman S, Teasdale J (1969) Aversion therapy and behavior disorders: An analysis. University of Miami Press, Miami
Rasch W (1982) Angst vor der Abartigkeit. Über einen schwierigen Begriff der §§ 20, 21 StGB. Neue Z Strafrecht 5: 177

Raymond MJ (1956) A case of fetishism treated by aversion therapy. Br Med J II: 854
Raymond MJ (1969) Aversion therapy for sexual deviations. Br J Psychiatry 115: 979
Reinecker H (1978) Selbstkontrolle: Verhaltenstherapeutische und kognitive Grundlagen, Techniken und Therapiemethoden. Müller, Salzburg
Reitz W, Keil WE (1971) Behavioral treatment of an exhibitionist. J Behav Ther Exp Psychiatry 2: 67
Rhodes RJ, Levinson M (1977) Sexual deviancy, treatment: A case study of a child molester. J Kans Med Soc 78: 122
Rieber J, Meyer AE, Schmidt G, Schorsch E, Sigusch V (1976) Stellungnahme zu stereotaktischen Hirnoperationen an Menschen mit abweichendem Sexualverhalten. Sexualmed 5: 442
Riemann F (1968) Psychoanalyse der Perversionen. Z Psychosom Med 14: 3
Robertiello RC (1971) A more positive view of perversions. Psychoanal Rev 58: 3
Rooth FG, Marks JM (1974) Persistent exhibitionism: Short term response to aversion, self-regulation and relaxation treatments. Arch Sex Behav 3: 227
Rosen RC, Kopel SA (1977) Penile plethysmography and biofeedback in the treatment of a transvestite-exhibitionist. J Consult Clin Psychol 45: 908
Rosenthal TI (1973) Response-contingent versus fixed punishment in aversion conditioning of pedophilia: A case study. J Nerv Ment Dis 156: 440
Sachs J (1965) Die Behandlung von Sexualdelinquenten in Dänemark. Beitr Sexualforsch 34: 69
Schmieschek H (1977) Verhaltenstherapie bei sexuellen Deviationen. Psychiatr Neurol Med Psychol (Leipz) 29: 725
Schorsch E (1971) Sexualstraftäter. Enke, Stuttgart
Schorsch E, Becker N (1977) Angst, Lust, Zerstörung. Sadismus als soziales und kriminelles Handeln. Zur Psychodynamik sexueller Tötungen. Rowohlt, Reinbek
Schorsch E, Schmidt G (1979) Hypothalamotomie bei sexuellen Abweichungen. Eine Kritik aus sexualwissenschaftlicher Sicht. Nervenarzt 50: 689
Schwartz MF, Masters WH (1983) Conceptual factors in the treatment of paraphilias: A preliminary report. J Sex Marital Ther 9: 3
Seiderer-Hartig M (1977) Verhaltenstherapie bei Fetischismus ohne Aversionstechniken. Partnerberatung 14: 36
Seiderer-Hartig M (1980) Die Rolle des Therapeuten und die therapeutische Beziehung in der Verhaltenstherapie. In: Petzold H (Hrsg) Die Rolle des Therapeuten und die therapeutische Beziehung. Junfermann, Paderborn
Serber M (1970) Shame aversion therapy. J Behav Ther Exp Psychiatry 1: 213
Serber M (1972) Shame aversion therapy with and without heterosexual retraining. In: Rubin SE, Franks CM (eds) Advances in behavior therapy. Academic Press, New York
Sigusch V (1977) Medizinische Experimente am Menschen. Das Beispiel Psychochirurgie. Jahrbuch für kritische Medizin (Beilage zum Argument-Sonderband AS 17). Argument-Verlag, Berlin
Sigusch V (1978) Die Kastration des Mannes. Sexualmed 7: 984
Sigusch V (1980) Therapie sexueller Störungen, 2. Aufl. Thieme, Stuttgart
Sigusch V (Hrsg) (1982) Die sexuelle Frage. Konkret, Hamburg
Sigusch V (1984) Vom Trieb und von der Liebe. Campus, Frankfurt New York
Snaith RP, Collins SA (1981) Five exhibitionists and a method of treatment. Br J Psychiatry 138: 126
Socarides CW (1959) Meaning and content of a pedophiliac perversion. J Am Psychoanal Assoc 7: 84
Socarides CW (1960) The development of a fetishistic perversion. J Am Psychoanal Assoc 8: 281
Statistisches Bundesamt Wiesbaden (1981) Rechtspflege. Reihe 3: Strafverfolgung 1980. Kohlhammer, Stuttgart Mainz
Stevenson J, Jones IH (1972) Behavior therapy technique for exhibitionism. Arch Gen Psychiatry 27: 839

Stevenson J, Wolpe J (1960) Recovery from sexual deviations through overcoming non-sexual neurotic responses. Am J Psychiatry 116: 737
Stoller RJ (1968) Sex and gender. Science House, New York, Hogarth, London
Stoller RJ (1975) Perversion: The erotic form of hatred. Random House, New York
Stolorow RD (1979) Psychosexuality and the representational world. Int J Psychoanal 60: 39
Stolorow RD, Grand H (1973) A partial analysis of a perversion involving bugs. Int J Psychoanal 54: 349
Strupp H, Luborsky L (eds) (1962) Research in psychotherapy. American Psychological Association, Washington
Stürup GK (1963) Die Behandlung der Sexualkriminalität in Skandinavien. In: Bauer F (Hrsg) Sexualität und Verbrechen. Fischer, Frankfurt
Stuhr U (1984) Deutungsarbeit im psychoanalytischen Dialog. Beiheft zu "Materialien zur Psychoanalyse und analytisch orientierten Psychotherapie". Vandenhoek u. Ruprecht, Göttingen
Thomä H, Kächele H (1973) Wissenschaftstheoretische und methodologische Probleme der klinisch psychoanalytischen Forschung. Psyche (Stuttg) 27: 203, 309
Thorpe JG et al. (1964) Aversion relief therapy: A new method for general application. Behav Res Ther 2: 71
Van Deventer AD, Laws DR (1978) Orgasmic reconditioning to redirect sexual arousal in pedophiles. Behav Res Ther 9: 748
Wälder R (1936) The principle of multiple function: observations on over-determination. Psychoanal Q 5: 45-62
Wardlaw GR, Miller PJ (1978) A controlled exposure technique in the elimination of exhibitionism. J Behav Ther Exp Psychiatry 8: 27
Wickramasekera J (1977) Aversion behavior rehearsal for sexual exhibitionism. J Behav Ther Exp Psychiatry 8: 135
Wijesinghe B (1977) Massed aversion treatment for sexual deviance. J Behav Ther Exp Psychiatry 8: 135
Winnicott DW (1958) Through pediatrics to psychoanalysis. Basic Books, New York
Wishart D (1978) Clustan user manual. Edinburgh
Wittmann L (1981) Verhaltenstherapie und Psychodynamik. Beltz, Weinheim Basel
Wolpe J (1958) Psychotherapy by reciprocal inhibition. Stanford University Press, Stanford
Yates AJ (1970) Behavior therapy. Wiley, New York

GPSR Compliance

The European Union's (EU) General Product Safety Regulation (GPSR) is a set of rules that requires consumer products to be safe and our obligations to ensure this.

If you have any concerns about our products, you can contact us on ProductSafety@springernature.com

In case Publisher is established outside the EU, the EU authorized representative is:

Springer Nature Customer Service Center GmbH
Europaplatz 3
69115 Heidelberg, Germany

Batch number: 10704713

Printed by Printforce, the Netherlands